SURGERY - PROCEDURES, COMPLICATIONS, AND RESULTS

BARIATRIC SURGERY

PREVALENCE, COMPLICATIONS AND IMPACT ON QUALITY OF LIFE

SURGERY - PROCEDURES, COMPLICATIONS, AND RESULTS

Additional books in this series can be found on Nova's website under the Series tab.

Additional e-books in this series can be found on Nova's website under the e-book tab.

SURGERY - PROCEDURES, COMPLICATIONS, AND RESULTS

BARIATRIC SURGERY

PREVALENCE, COMPLICATIONS AND IMPACT ON QUALITY OF LIFE

MANDY CHAMBERS
EDITOR

New York

Library of Congress Cataloging-in-Publication Data

ISBN: 978-1-63463-697-1
Library of Congress Control Number: 2014957690

Published by Nova Science Publishers, Inc. † New York

Contents

Preface **vii**

Chapter 1 Optimal Physical Activity and Exercise Following Bariatric Surgery **1**
Matthew D. Barberio, PhD, Rosemary Lu, BS and Monica J. Hubal, PhD

Chapter 2 Small Intestinal Bacterial Overgrowth after Bariatric Surgery **19**
Iman Andalib, MD, Naveen Gara, MD, Bikram S. Bal, MD, Timothy R. Shope, MD and Timothy R. Koch, MD

Chapter 3 Complications of Bariatric Surgery, Improvement of Comorbidities and Impact on Quality of Life **35**
Jaime Ruiz-Tovar, MD, PhD and Carolina Llavero

Chapter 4 Long Term Diabetes Outcomes After Bariatric Surgery **61**
Richard W. Carroll, Jeremy D. Krebs and Rinki Murphy

Chapter 5 Adjustable Gastric Banding Surgery: Impact on Inflammation and Iron Metabolism **85**
Cristina Catarino, Susana Coimbra, Luís Belo, Luís Monteiro, Elísio Costa and Alice Santos-Silva

Chapter 6 Pregnancy After Bariatric Surgery **107**
Catarina Policiano, Alexandre Valentim Lourenço, Luísa Pinto and Luís Mendes Graça

Chapter 7 Anesthesia Consideration and Management for Bariatric Surgery **121**
Antoni Sabaté, MD, PhD and Sandra Llaurado, MD

Index **131**

Preface

In response to rapidly increasing rates of obesity, bariatric weight loss surgeries have increased worldwide, reaching approximately 341,000 procedures in 2011. Bariatric surgery is a major medical intervention with the primary goals of chronically reducing excess weight loss, decreasing incidence and severity of obesity related co-morbidities, and overall improvement in quality of life. Despite widespread evidence of bariatric surgery effectiveness on excess weight loss and resolution of co-morbidities, the effects of weight loss surgery on overall cardiorespiratory fitness and physical activity levels (two critical components of overall health) have yet to be defined. This book discusses the prevalence of bariatric surgery, as well as the complications and it's impact on quality of life.

Chapter 1 – Bariatric surgery typically results in health improvements across multiple obesity-related comorbidities, in addition to losses of excess weight. It is commonly believed that weight loss following surgery would improve physical activity (PA) levels as movement becomes less difficult, resulting in increased cardiorespiratory (CR) fitness. Increased physical activity levels post-surgery would help optimize and sustain weight loss and other co-morbidity improvements. However, evaluation of fitness and PA levels after surgery-induced weight loss is a nascent field without consensus about the efficacy of current surgical programs to evoke increased fitness and PA changes. Few studies to date have measured changes in different types of fitness, from musculoskeletal function to cardiorespiratory endurance. Furthermore, the limited available research suggesting significant increases in self-reported physical activity following surgery have used objective PA measures, making interpretation difficult. The goal of this chapter is to review existing literature regarding fitness and PA changes following weight-loss surgery. As part of this goal, we will briefly review some basic tenets of physical fitness related to activity and exercise. We will also relate fitness and PA changes to sustained weight-loss and reduced health risks following surgery. Finally, we will highlight gaps in the literature and suggest specific research topics needed to address these relationships, so that optimal bariatric surgery programs can be designed to maximize improvements in fitness.

Chapter 2 – Worldwide, the prevalence of obesity continues to rise. Attempts at modification of diet and lifestyle often fail to prevent the medical complications of obesity. Bariatric surgery is being increasingly utilized for treatment of obesity. Despite being a gold standard therapy for management of medically-complicated obesity, bariatric surgery has been associated with multiple complications including nutritional deficiencies, bloating, and dyspepsia. Ongoing clinical research has shown that bariatric surgery can lead to postoperative small intestinal bacterial overgrowth with its related nutritional deficiencies. Bacterial overgrowth may result from alteration of the host defense mechanisms, including loss of gastric acid or diminished exposure to bile acids, and altered upper gastrointestinal motility. Other co-morbid disorders, including diabetes mellitus, chronic narcotic use, use of proton pump inhibitors and antidepressants appear to play a role in the development of bacterial overgrowth. Although microbial investigation of jejunal aspirates is the gold standard for detecting bacterial overgrowth, glucose-hydrogen breath testing is increasingly becoming the test of choice for this diagnosis. The treatment for bacterial overgrowth can be very challenging and can include treatment of the underlying disease, correction of vitamin deficiencies, and discontinuation of motility-altering medications. Antibiotics are effective, but only a few studies concerning choice of and duration of antibiotic therapy exist. Herein, we describe the potential mechanisms for the development of small intestinal bacterial overgrowth, the effects of bacterial overgrowth on nutrients, the methods of diagnosis of bacterial overgrowth, and treatment options for this disorder.

Chapter 3 – More than 2/3 of the U.S, population is overweight or obese. Obesity is on the rise and the incidence is increasing most rapidly in the morbidly obese population, i.e. those with a BMIs exceeding 40 kg/m^2. Epidemiological studies estimate the prevalence of morbid obesity around 0.5%, but this rate is probably underestimated, as many morbidly obese subjects are not under any medical control. Only surgery results in substantial, long-term weight loss for obese individuals. Therefore, the performance of bariatric procedure has increased exponentially in the last 2 decades; from less than 9,000 procedures in 1993 to a high of over 115,000 in 2004. Actually, the number of bariatric procedures performed is even higher.

Despite nowadays most bariatric techniques are performed laparoscopically, the complications rate still represents a challenge for many surgeons. Complications associated to these approaches are often life-threatening conditions. Morbidly obese patients are high risk subjects and therefore, bariatric surgery must be considered a high risk procedure though the patients are operated for a benign condition. Complications include medical (deep vein thrombosis, pulmonary embolism, atelectasia, pneumonia,..) and surgical items (anastomotic leak, bleeding, surgical site infection,…).

Even considering the surgical risk, bariatric surgery has demonstrated much more advantages than disadvantages. Bariatric surgery can solve many comorbidities, such as diabetes mellitus, hypertension, dyslipidemia, pulmonary disorders, osteoarthritis,…, and reduces significantly the risk of developing new health problems, such as cardiovascular or neoplastic events. Altogether, this leads to a significant improvement of the quality of life. The patients feel healthier and this has a positive psychological impact. There are many scales available to evaluate quality of life, but all of them coincide in that bariatric surgery achieves a significant improvement in the quality of life of morbidly obese patients.

Chapter 4 – Bariatric surgery was developed primarily as a therapy to induce weight loss. Indeed, those with type 2 diabetes were originally not considered surgical candidates due to the perceived high risk nature of surgery in these individuals. However, significant post-operative improvements in diabetes control were noted early in the history of bariatric surgery. Multiple retrospective and prospective studies have since supported this finding, including a number of high quality randomised trials. Variable definitions of diabetes outcomes are used within the published literature complicating comparative analysis. This chapter will review the published literature on glycaemic outcomes at least 12 months following bariatric surgery, and discuss the importance of a consistent set of definitions when reporting on diabetes outcomes.

Chapter 5 – Obesity is increasing all over the world both in developed and underdeveloped countries and is known to be associated with inflammatory changes, insulin resistance and with a hyperlipidemic state. The adipocyte is an important source of adipokines, such as adiponectin, leptin, interleukin (IL)-6 and tumor necrosis factor alpha, and their levels are significantly altered in the plasma of obese patients. Some of these adipokines are known to be associated with dyslipidemia, insulin resistance, vascular dysfunction, and inflammation, and seem to contribute to the development of cardiovascular disease (CVD). Moreover, some inflammatory markers, such as C-reactive protein (CRP), show an independent positive association with body mass index (BMI), and with increased CVD risk. Cardiovascular morbidity and mortality is associated with the classic risk factors, dyslipidemia, hypertension and impaired glucose metabolism. More recently, inflammatory mechanisms have been accepted as important players in the development of atherosclerotic vascular disease. Obesity, an inflammatory condition, is also an important CVD risk factor.

Recently, it was found that the adipose tissue also expresses hepcidin, and, therefore, may have a direct involvement in iron metabolism. Indeed, obesity is also known to be associated with iron deficiency. The synthesis of hepcidin, an acute phase protein that regulates iron availability, is enhanced in obesity, through IL-6 and leptin secretion by adipose tissue, and may lead to iron deficiency. Gastric band surgery is a safe surgical procedure for the treatment of morbid obesity, almost without mortality in the perioperative period and a low long-term mortality rate from unrelated causes. Using laparoscopic surgery a gradual, continuous and well-programmed weight loss, is achieved, as well as, a post-operative increasing quality of life and the co-morbidities associated with obesity are also reduced in 75% of patients. In this book chapter, we will focus on the relationship between obesity, adipose tissue, inflammation and iron metabolism, and we will discuss the impact of gastric banding in the cross-talk between these important factors in obesity.

Chapter 6 – Obesity rates and its serious comorbidities have been rising worldwide resulting in a significant loss of life expectancy. Women of reproductive age are generally healthy and metabolic disorders in this age group are uncommon. However they account for a large group of the obese population and pre-pregnancy Body Mass Index (BMI) has been strongly associated with an increased risk of diabetes, hypertension and dyslipidemia, not only during pregnancy but also in the following decades of life. Pre-pregnancy overweight and obesity are also independent risk factors for serious comorbid cardiovascular events (ischemic heart disease, cardiac heart failure) even in the absence of metabolic syndrome.

Chapter 7 – Morbidly obese patients are already at high risk for cardiovascular and respiratory functional overload related to varying degrees of metabolic syndrome. Most of patients request for bariatric surgery in an early stage of the disease, therefore low rates of mortality and morbidity are the standard. Even that, perioperative complications are related to previous comorbidity, age, body mass index and type of bariatric surgery. Restrictive procedures are not expected to have mortality, but all complication rates are 3.2%, and readmission rate is 4.3%. For gastric bypass procedures, the complication rate is 16%, the readmission rate of 6.6% and mortality around 0.4%, which account intra operatively in 0.18%. of patients. Consequently, anesthetic management of morbid obese patients is a challenge, even to an experienced anesthesiologist and to do that effectively, these key points have to be considered.

In: Bariatric Surgery
Editor: Mandy Chambers

ISBN: 978-1-63463-697-1

Chapter 1

Optimal Physical Activity and Exercise Following Bariatric Surgery

Matthew D. Barberio, PhD, Rosemary Lu, BS, and Monica J. Hubal*, PhD

Department of Integrative Systems Biology
George Washington University School of Medicine
Research Center for Genetic Medicine
Children's National Medical Center, Washington, DC, US

Abstract

Bariatric surgery typically results in health improvements across multiple obesity-related comorbidities, in addition to losses of excess weight. It is commonly believed that weight loss following surgery would improve physical activity (PA) levels as movement becomes less difficult, resulting in increased cardiorespiratory (CR) fitness. Increased physical activity levels post-surgery would help optimize and sustain weight loss and other co-morbidity improvements. However, evaluation of fitness and PA levels after surgery-induced weight loss is a nascent field without consensus about the efficacy of current surgical programs to evoke increased fitness and PA changes. Few studies to date have measured changes in different types of fitness, from musculoskeletal function to cardiorespiratory endurance. Furthermore, the limited available research suggesting significant increases in self-reported physical activity following surgery have used objective PA measures, making interpretation difficult. The goal of this chapter is to review existing literature regarding fitness and PA changes following weight-loss surgery. As part of this goal, we will briefly review some basic tenets of physical fitness related to activity and exercise. We will also relate fitness and PA changes to sustained weight-loss and reduced health risks following surgery. Finally, we will highlight gaps in the literature and suggest specific research topics needed to address these relationships, so that optimal bariatric surgery programs can be designed to maximize improvements in fitness.

* Telephone: 202.476.6296; Fax: 202.476.6014; Corresponding author. mhubal@childrensnational.org.

Glossary of Terms

Physical activity: Bodily movements produced by skeletal muscle that result in an increase in energy expenditure.

Exercise: A form of physical activity that is structured with planned sequences of repetitive body movements with the goal of maintenance or improvements in physical fitness.

Physical fitness: Ability to carry out daily tasks with vigor and alertness, without undue fatigue and with ample energy to enjoy leisure-time pursuits and to meet unforeseen emergencies

Overload: Physical activity and exercise that an individual is unaccustomed to presents a positive stressor to various physiological systems.

Adaptation: Molecular, structural, and mechanical changes in physiological systems so that subsequent stressors are adequately handled by the systems.

Injury: Damage done to various tissues or various physiological systems as a result of physical stress.

Cardiorespiratory fitness: The capability of circulatory and respiratory systems ability to deliver fuel during sustained physical activity and to remove metabolic waste products.

Muscular strength: The amount of external force a muscle or a muscle group can exert.

Muscular endurance: The ability of a muscle or muscle groups to repetitively produce external force without undue fatigue.

Body composition: The measurement of the relative amounts of body fat, lean tissue (i.e. muscle), bone, and other vital organs.

Flexibility: The ability to move a joint about its full range of motion.

Introduction

In response to rapidly increasing rates of obesity, bariatric weight loss surgeries have increased worldwide, reaching approximately 341,000 procedures in 2011 [1]. Bariatric surgery is a major medical intervention with the primary goals of chronically reducing excess weight loss, decreasing incidence and severity of obesity related co-morbidities, and overall improvement in quality of life. Despite widespread evidence of bariatric surgery effectiveness on excess weight loss and resolution of co-morbidities, the effects of weight loss surgery on overall cardiorespiratory fitness and physical activity levels (two critical components of overall health) have yet to be defined.

Increased physical activity is associated with reduced incidences of chronic disease and all-cause mortality [2-4]. Physical activity generally improves overall physical fitness, including its underlying components, including cardiorespiratory, muscular, and metabolic fitness, though specific benefits will vary based on the type and amount of activities done.

While the main goal of weight loss surgery is the reduction of excess weight, improvements in other lifestyle choices (such as physical activity levels) are essential to overall improvements in quality of life [5]. Despite this, very little research is available regarding post-operative improvements in physical fitness or the various components that make up overall physical fitness [6]. A key remaining question is the identification of independent and interactive effects of surgery and weight loss on cardiorespiratory fitness? Another question is whether spontaneous physical activity increases following substantial weight loss. Further investigations regarding changes in physical fitness following surgery are needed for the appropriate exercise prescription for the post-operative populations.

Physical activity plays vital roles in long term excess weight loss and improvements in quality of life following surgery. In previous investigations, those considered to be morbidly obese cite reductions in mobility and physical activity, as a negative impact of their excess weight [7]. This reduced PA can compound the obese state by further reducing energy expenditure. Increased physical activity can positively impact outcomes following weight loss surgery by elevating energy balance both acutely (i.e. during physical activity) and chronically (i.e. elevated resting metabolic rate, maintenance of lean body mass, etc.). However, investigations into the ability of weight loss surgeries to result in improvements in physical activity levels are scarce and inconclusive. Additionally, investigations into optimal strategies for structured/prescribed physical activity recommendations in the weight loss surgery population are lacking.

The purpose of this chapter is to first provide a short primer on fitness and physical activity, followed by a summarization of the literature to date regarding changes in cardiorespiratory fitness and physical activity following bariatric surgery. We will also highlight relationships between enhanced physical activity and fitness and reductions in health risks and obesity related co-morbidities. Finally, we will identify specific areas that warrant further investigation to better understand the relationships between weight loss surgery and improvements in overall health.

Excess Weight Loss Efficacy following Bariatric Surgery

Most recent estimates indicate that approximately 341,000 metabolic/bariatric surgical procedures occurred worldwide in 2011, of which the Roux-ex-Y gastric bypass (RYGB) accounted for 47%, sleeve gastrectomy (SG) 28%, adjustable gastric banding (AGB) 18%, and biliopancreatic diversion/duodenal switch (BPD/DS) 2.2% of total procedures [1]. These values are estimated from voluntary survey participation of over 50 countries/regions represented in the International Federation for Surgery of Obesity and Metabolic Disorders (IFSO) and may under-represent precise totals.

The most recognizable goal of weight loss surgery is to induce chronic reductions in excess weight, defined as the difference between preoperative weight and the ideal weight and often represented as a percentage (% excess weight loss = (weight lost/ preoperative excess weight)*100). The most recent meta-analysis of available data (1990 – 2004) indicates that patients lost an average of 61.2% of excess weight following surgery, regardless of the type of procedure performed [8]. Resolution of obesity related comorbidities in patients following surgery were as follows: 76.8% diabetes; 61.7% hypertension; 85.7% sleep apnea and; hyperlipidemia improved in 70% of patients, regardless of procedure type [8]. There is significant variance in these outcomes based on procedure. We refer readers to Buchwald et al. (2004) for a more complete analysis of the successes of individual procedure types. It is important to point out that most (if not all) of these co-morbidities are also significantly affected by physical activity, meaning that resolution following surgery is affected both by surgery and each patient's physical activity pattern.

While it is has widely been shown that bariatric weight loss surgery is successful in acutely reducing excess weight, a growing concern regarding long-term (> 5 yrs.) excess weight reduction and maintenance exists, as well as interest in long-term health improvements [9-11]. A key debate in this area is whether co-morbidity resolution is weight-loss dependent or independent, and to what extent resolution is driven by weight loss itself. As long-term weight loss is augmented by adopting positive lifestyle strategies following surgery, research in fitness and PA changes post-surgery are essential to the success of bariatric surgery programs.

Physical Activity, Exercise, and Physical Fitness

Before moving on to review the literature on fitness and PA changes following surgery, we feel it is beneficial to provide a short primer on exercise physiology for the current reader. Physical activity and physical fitness have been defined and discussed in detail previously, but here we seek to briefly discuss and summarize these key concepts [12, 13].

Physical fitness is defined as "the ability to carry out daily tasks with vigor and alertness, without undue fatigue and with ample energy to enjoy leisure-time pursuits and to meet unforeseen emergencies" [12]. Evidence overwhelmingly supports a positive relationship between physical fitness levels and health-related risks factors [3]. *Physical activity* is defined as bodily movements produced by skeletal muscle that results in an increase in energy expenditure [12]. Physical activity encompasses many day-to-day activities (such as walking or cooking), as well as participation in planned events such as recreational sports. *Exercise* is a specific form of physical activity that is structured with planned sequences of repetitive body movements with the goal of maintenance or improvements in physical fitness [14].

Physically-active lifestyles delay all-cause mortality, as well as reduce the risk of developing Type 2 diabetes mellitus, coronary heart disease, and multiple forms of cancer [4]. Evidence largely supports a dose-response relationship between the amount of physical activity and health-related outcomes [4, 15], though data regarding the quantities of physical activity required for such benefits is not clear and is likely specific to each outcome. Most large epidemiological studies have found that a minimum of approximately 150 $min \cdot wk^{-1}$ (~1000 $kilocalories \cdot wk^{-1}$) is sufficient for health-related benefits [3]. However, few studies have addressed this PA level cutoff, and other lifestyle interventions, in severely obese populations [16].

Physical fitness cannot be described as a singular phenotype, but instead can be divided into five health-related components that can be individually evaluated [3, 17]. Below we discuss the five health-related components of physical fitness, describe how they are clinically evaluated, and note the impact of a physically active lifestyle on each component. For the purposes of this chapter, we will focus most heavily on cardiorespiratory fitness.

Principals of Training and Adaptation

Before discussing the health-related components of physical fitness, it is important to note the basic principles underlying how physical activity and exercise improve physical fitness. The general adaptation syndrome, developed by Dr. Hans Selye, describes three stages of a stress response: alarm and reaction, development of resistance, and finally exhaustion [18]. This model is easily applied to physical activity and exercise to describe how they promote health improvement:

Overload (alarm and reaction) – physical activity and exercise that an individual is unaccustomed to presents a positive stressor to various physiological systems.

Adaptation (resistance development) – continual overload applied to a system results in adaptations (i.e. molecular, structural, and mechanical) so that subsequent stressors are adequately handled by the system.

Injury (exhaustion) – if the overload of the applied stressors from physical activity and exercise is too great or the appropriate adaptations have not occurred, then injuries such as muscle strains, ligament tears, and bone fracturing may result.

Providing adequate overload (without going so far as to evoke a significant injury response) to physiological systems is essential to promotion of positive beneficial adaptations of these systems. Physical activity and exercise have the benefit of being quantifiable and easily adjusted so that the appropriate stressor is achieved and risk of injury reduced. For instance, the intensity of an exercise is easily changed by adjusting the pace (i.e. intensity) at which one walks or runs, while in resistance training the amount of resistance used can be increased or decreased. Another important variable in determining overload is the amount (i.e. dose) of any given physical activity or exercise that is performed. This is easily change by altering the amount of time spent doing any particular endurance exercise or by decreasing the amount of repetitions during resistance training. Lastly, the frequency at which one participates in any form of physical activity is important to determining the amount of overload that is applied.

A final important principle for physical activity and exercise is specificity. The principle of specificity states that all adaptations will be specific to the applied stressor. Thus, it is important that any exercise or physical activity be planned in accordance with the outcome goal. For instance, if increased muscular strength is desired, resistance-type exercise as opposed to endurance training is indicated. Later in this chapter, we will discuss the recommended amounts, intensities, and frequency of exercise and physical activity to promote health and well-being for specific health-related components following intervention such as surgery.

Cardiorespiratory Fitness

Cardiorespiratory fitness is defined as the capability of circulatory and respiratory systems ability to deliver energy during sustained physical activity and to remove metabolic waste products [12]. Alternatively, it may also be defined as the ability to sustain moderate-to-high intensity exercise for prolonged periods of time [14]. Traditionally, maximal cardiorespiratory fitness has been determined by a maximal progressive incremental exercise test performed on a cycle ergometer or treadmill, in which the maximal rate of oxygen consumption (VO_{2max}; ml $O_2 \cdot kg^{-1}$ body mass $\cdot$ min^{-1}) is measured by indirect calorimetry. It may also be predicted by the utilization of a submaximal exercise test from which the results are extrapolated to estimate maximal ability [14] via equation.

Regular moderate-vigorous physical activity and exercise result in increased cardiorespiratory fitness [3]. Current recommendations of the American College of Sports Medicine (ACSM), American Heart Association (AHA), and the *2008 Physical Activity Guidelines for Americans* prescribe at least 30 $min{\cdot}d^{-1}$ of moderate intensity exercise on at least 5 $d{\cdot}wk^{-1}$ [15, 19, 20]. Research also indicates that more vigorous physical activity requires less time and results in similar, and potentially greater, cardiorespiratory benefits [3], though this relationship will be specific to each element underlying cardiorespiratory fitness.

Routine participation in cardiorespiratory exercise (also commonly referred to as aerobic or endurance exercise training) results in various physiological adaptations in the heart, vasculature, and skeletal muscle that promote increases in cardiorespiratory fitness. One major structural change that occurs during training is an increase in the volume of the left ventricle. This adaptation reduces the energetic costs of the heart by increasing stroke volume, reducing resting heart rate, and reducing submaximal exercise heart rate.

Skeletal muscle also undergoes significant adaptations that promote an increase in cardiorespiratory fitness. First, an increase in vascularization of the skeletal muscle occurs as more capillaries form around individual fibers. This increase in capillarity results in a greater perfusion of the skeletal muscle, especially during exercise, increasing oxygen delivery to and extraction by the fibers. Skeletal muscle also undergoes various metabolic adaptations, including increase in mitochondrial content of the individual fibers, as well as increases in various key enzymes important for the uptake and oxidation of glucose and triglycerides.

Collectively, these adaptations are essential to the favorable changes that occur in various cardiometabolic risk factors that are associated with physical activity and exercise. Improvements in blood lipid profiles, reductions in insulin resistance, and reductions in systemic markers of inflammation have routinely been found as a result of regular physical activity, independent of weight loss [3].

Muscular Strength & Endurance

Muscular strength and muscle endurance have been combined to describe muscular fitness [13]. *Muscular strength* is related to the amount of external force a muscle or a muscle group can exert. Standard measurement of muscular strength requires the use of dynamometers or tensiometers to measure force produced during an isometric (non-shortening) contraction. Other tests, such as a 1-repition maximum (1-RM) are more commonly used to determine this value, and measure dynamic, rather than static, strength. The 1-RM is defined as "the greatest resistance that can be moved through a full range of motion in a controlled manner" [14]. Muscular strength should always be measured in the muscle group of interest to a particular task. *Muscular endurance* is defined as the ability of a muscle or muscle groups to repetitively produce external force without undue fatigue. The standard of measure is through use of isokinetic dynamometer, but is more often determined through tests such as sit-ups, sit-and-stand, push-ups, and pull-ups. Dynamic tests using free weights may also be used to determined absolute muscular endurance (total number of repetitions at a given resistance) or the relative muscular endurance (total number of repetitions at a resistance equal to percentage of 1-RM).

Resistance training promotes skeletal muscle hypertrophy and increased skeletal muscle fiber size through an increase in protein synthesis. Resultant increases in muscle fiber size and fiber density result in an increased muscular strength and muscular endurance. This also can result in increased lean body mass and a greater percentage of lean body mass to overall mass. Regular resistance training can also result in increased neural motor unit firing rates, recruitment of higher threshold motor units, and more synchronous motor unit firing [21]. In fact, these neural adaptations are largely responsible for early increases in muscular strength and endurance, as individuals adapt to the complex movements of resistance training.

Because adaptation is specific to the applied exercise stressor, strategies to promote muscular strength and muscular endurance are distinct. For promoting increases in muscular endurance the American College of Sports Medicine (ACSM) recommends a minimum of 10-15 repetitions for each major muscle group 2-3 days per week ($d{\cdot}wk^{-1}$) [17]. For increases in muscular strength, it is recommended that a minimum of 1-3 sets consisting of 8-12 repetitions at 70-85% of 1-RM be performed 2-3 $d{\cdot}wk^{-1}$[17]. It is important to progressively increase the resistance so that a continual overload is applied to the muscle as adaptations occur. Resistance training can be completed through the use of specialized machinery, which assists movements, or free weights, and the choice of equipment should be based on experience level of the individual.

Body Composition

Another component of fitness is *body composition;* defined as the measurement of the relative amounts of body fat, lean tissue (i.e. muscle), bone, and other vital organs. These values are all obtainable through dual-energy X-ray absorptiometry (DEXA) or other scanning technologies. However, other more cost- and time-effective measurements (such as multiple site skinfolds and body mass index) are more commonly used as indices of body composition. Skinfolds assume that approximately 1/3 of all body fat is located subcutaneously, but this is largely influenced by race, ethnicity, and age [22]. To account for these variables, specific regression equations can be used to determine the percentage of body fat from skinfolds [23], though anthropomorphic equations always contain some amount of error. Body mass index (BMI) is a commonly used calculation to assess body mass (in kg) relative to height (in meters) of an individual. Naturally, the calculated BMI values cannot distinguish between lean body mass and fat mass, but a BMI $\geq 30\ kg{\cdot}m^2$ is associated with an increase in health related risk factors [24].

Flexibility

Flexibility is also a component of overall fitness and is defined as the ability to move a joint about its full range of motion [12, 14]. Flexibility can be separated into two specific types: static and dynamic. Static flexibility is ability to reach a specific point in the range of motion of a joint whereas dynamic flexibility is the ability to move quickly throughout the entire range of motion without resistance [21]. Good flexibility is an important to improving quality of life and mitigating join pain and injuries, especially in aging populations.

Standard laboratory methods are used to determine flexibility, measured in degrees, through the use of goniometers. Less accurate methodology using tape-measures (i.e. sit and reach tests) are often used to evaluate flexibility at the hip clinically [14]. Just as muscular strength is specific to muscle groups, flexibility is joint specific and can be influenced by joint type and muscle "tightness" [14].

Here we have introduced and briefly discussed physical fitness, the underlying health-related components of physical fitness, and some standard measurement procedures. For more thorough discussion regarding these topics, we suggest you consult the appropriate citations or exercise science textbooks. For the purposes of this chapter, we will now focus mainly on the effects bariatric weight loss surgery's effect on changes in cardiorespiratory outcomes.

Bariatric Weight Loss Surgery, Cardiorespiratory Fitness, and Physical Activity

Low cardiorespiratory fitness results in increased incidences of cardiovascular disease, all-cause mortality, and an increased relative risk of death similar to those associated with diabetes and tobacco use [2, 9, 25-31]. Furthermore, post-surgery complications and 30-day readmission rates were significantly related to cardiorespiratory fitness levels prior to surgery [32]. However, very few studies have analyzed changes in cardiorespiratory fitness following surgery. Also concerning is evidence that a significant portion (~30%) of weight loss may be due to loss of fat free mass [33, 34]. In the following section, we will discuss the limited available evidence regarding changes in cardiorespiratory fitness, changes in physical activity fitness, and the relationship between long-term weight loss and physical activity following weight loss surgery.

Does Weight Loss Surgery Result Enhance Cardiorespiratory Fitness?

de Souza et al. (2010) showed that VO_{2max} was significantly increased (22.1 ± 2.1 vs. 15.8 ± 2.1 ml· $kg^{-1}\cdot min^{-1}$) 12 months following RYGBP. Reductions in BMI in this cohort were also significantly correlated to exercise capacity [6]. To date, this is the only investigation to study bariatric surgery and changes in cardiorespiratory fitness through indirect calorimetry. Leite et al. (2013) found similar results using the six-minute walk (6MWT), an indirect surrogate for cardiorespiratory fitness in which individuals walk for 6 minutes and try to cover as much distance as possible. Sixty-five individuals who had undergone surgery in the previous 24 months and had a current BMI < 30 kg/m^2 covered similar distances in the 6MWT to that of non-obese controls and significantly more than individuals who had undergone surgery but were still considered obese with a BMI > 30 kg/m^2 [35]. Similar results were found by Varga et al. (2013), in which reduction in BMI correlated with significantly increased 6MWT three months following surgery [36].

Interestingly, two studies by the same group have studied the effect of weight loss surgery on functional measures of pulmonary function. Only one study found an increased lung volume (3.5%), increased expiratory reserve volume (88.9%), and decreased inspiratory reserve volume (-20.4%) 12 months following RYGBP [35, 37]. More controlled analyses will be required, but these data indicate that bariatric weight loss surgery may result in significant positive cardiorespiratory benefits.

Does Weight Loss Surgery Result in Spontaneous Increases in Physical Activity?

Reduction in weight following surgery presents the opportunity for individuals to increase physical activity levels, as physical limitations are eased. Available evidence indicates that patients routinely report increased levels of physical activity through the use of various lifestyle questionnaires (Table 1). However, self-reporting physical activity levels using questionnaires was recently brought into question by Bond et al. (2010). Their investigation found that patients significantly over-estimated the amount of time spent doing moderate-to-vigorous physical activity (MVPA; defined as a metabolic equivalent (MET) ≥ 3) and compliance (55% vs. 5%) with the recommended 150 $min \cdot wk^{-1}$ of physical activity when reported levels were compared to the use of accelerometers [38], which provide objective measures of PA.

Evidence from Structured Exercise Interventions Following Weight Loss Surgery

Even though these findings regarding over reporting are concerning, reported increases in post-operative physical activity levels have been associated with enhanced outcomes. A recent meta-analysis of 17 observational studies by Egberts et al. (2011) found that increased post-operative physical activity resulted in an average of 3.62 kg greater weight loss than those who had minimal physical activity. Of these 17 survey studies, 15 showed a positive relationship between physical activity levels and weight loss [52]. Mundi et al. (2013) and Josbeno et al. (2011) both found MVPA levels to be greater in those who lost ≥ 50% excess weight from pre-surgery baseline. Other studies have found that self-reported levels of physical activity have been associated with successful weight loss [40, 43-45, 47, 53, 54], BMI reductions [40, 41, 50], decreased fat mass [50], and increased lean body mass [50]. Even in patients who have regained a significant amount of weight, physical activity has been associated with lower long-term weight regain [10]. It is likely that altered physical activity levels, along with other lifestyle modifications such as nutritional and psychosocial, play a crucial role in maximizing the long-term success of post-operative excess weight loss. Future objective studies that explore whether bariatric weight loss surgery leads to spontaneous increases in regular physical activity will be crucial to understanding the role of physical activity in successful long-term weight loss.

Table 1. Effect of Physical Activity on Bariatric Weight-loss Surgery Outcomes

Study		Surgery Type	Prescribed or Spontaneous	Physical Activity Reporting	Follow-up Duration (mo)	% EWL	P-value	ΔBMI (kg/m^2)	P-value
Boan et al. 2004	[39]	RYGBP	Spontaneous	BQA	6	26.7[¥]	<0.0001	-14.0	<0.0001
Bond et al. 2004	[40]	GBP Control	Spontaneo-us	Self-report	24	68.2 ± 17.4	<0.0081[∞]	-31.5	0.0011[∞]
			Sedentary	Self-report	24	63.9 ± 19.5		-33.0	
Silver et al. 2006	[41]	RYGBP	Spontaneous	BRFSS	24.2 ± 7.9	55.8 ± 15.2[€]	N/A	N/A	N/A
Mathus-Vliegen and de Wit 2007	[42]	LAGB & OAGB	Spontaneous	HRQL	12	42.1 ± 17.9	N/A	-11.5	<0.001
					30	42.2 ± 22.8	N/A	-11.6	<0.001
					60	41.6 ± 26.2	N/A	-11.4	<0.001
Welch et al. 2008[#]	[43]	RYGBP	Spontaneous	BSSQ	<6	35.9 ± 13.7	N/A	-17.5[§]	N/A
					6 to 12	50.8 ± 15.0			N/A
					12 to 18	66.9 ± 41.1	N/A		N/A
					>18	65.7 ± 16.6	N/A		N/A
Colles et al. 2008[#]	[44]	LAGB	Spontaneous	BPAQ	4	32.2 ± 13.0	NS	-6.0	<0.001
					12	50.0 ± 20.7	<0.001	-9.3	<0.001
Bond et al. 2009[#]	[45]	RYGBP	Spontaneous[£]	IPAG-short	12	71.5 ± 15.5	0.049	-18.9 ± 4.6	0.013
						69.8 ± 14.1		-18.3 ± 4.6	
						63.1 ± 16.6		-16.9 ± 4.2	
Livhits et al. 2010[#]	[46]	RYGBP	Spontaneous	IPAG-short	40.1 ± 15.3	52.6 ± 22.4	<0.01	N/A	N/A
Forbush et al. 2011[#]	[47]	RYGBP	Spontaneous	AAF	12	82.7 ± 27.3	<0.01	-17.6[§]	N/A
					24	82.7 ± 23.2			
					36	84.0 ± 24.0			
					48	77.8 ± 26.8			
					60	76.0 ± 20.8			
Shah et al. 2011[#]	[48]	RYGBP	Prescribed	Supervision	1.5	2.1[€]		N/A	N/A

Study	Surgery Type	Prescribed or Spontaneous	Physical Activity Reporting	Follow-up Duration (mo)	% EWL	P-value	ΔBMI (kg/m^2)	P-value
	and GB		and diary	3	4.2[€]	<0.01	N/A	N/A
	Control	N/A	N/A	1.5	1.8[€]		N/A	N/A
				3	4.7[€]	<0.01	N/A	N/A
Josbeno et al. [49] 2011[#]	RYGBP	Spontaneous	SWPro	24	72.8 ± 10.8	0.02	-19.8	N/A
				36	53.0 ± 17.6		-12.7	N/A
				48	60.1 ± 21.5		-14.4	N/A
				60	58.0 ± 28.4		-16.9	N/A
Freire et al. [10] 2012	RYGBP	Spontaneous	Self-report	<24	59.1 ± 20.3[§]	NS	-17.5	N/A
				25 to 60			-22.3	N/A
				>61			-17.1	N/A
Vatier et al. [50] 2012	RYGBP	Spontaneous	MAQ	6	25.9 ± 19.7[€]	<0.0001	-9.1	<0.0001
				12	37.1 ± 20.5[€]	<0.0001	-13.0	<0.0001
Mundi et al. [51] 2013[#]	Non-lap band	Spontaneous	IPAG-short	12	33.2 ± 9.4	<0.001	-14.3	0.001
					67.1 ± 8.8	<0.001	-15.2	

RYGBP; Roux-en-Y gastric bypass. GBP; Gastric bypass. LAGB; Laparoscopic adjustable gastric banding. OAGB; Open adjustable gastric banding. GB; Gastric banding. BQA; Baseline Questionnaire of Activity. BRFSS; Behavioral Risk Factor Surveillance System Questionnaire. HRQL; Health Related Quality of Life Questionnaire. BSSQ; Bariatric Surgery Self-Management Questionnaire. SF-36; Medical Outcomes Trust Short Form-36. BPAQ; Baecke Physical Activity Questionnaire. IPAG-short; International Physical Activity Questionnaire short form. AAF, Arizona Activity Frequency Questionnaire. MAQ, Modifiable Activity Questionnaire. SWPro; BodyMedia SenseWear® Pro armband. P values represent significance for pre to postoperative values unless otherwise noted. [∞] P value represents significance between physical activity group and sedentary group. [#] Study identified physical activity as a significant determinant of weight loss. [£] Study separated patients into inactive/active, active/active, inactive/inactive groups based on pre/post-surgery physical activity levels. [¥] Mean % total weight loss. [€] Mean of total absolute weight loss (kg). [§] Mean all time points combined.

While the previous section highlighted a lack of consensus about spontaneous PA changes with surgery, there is also a lack of consensus regarding routine structured exercise. Routine structured PA is largely considered to be beneficial to overall health outcomes for the general population, though very few studies have examined appropriate strategies for severely obese populations and post-surgical patients [16, 55-57]. Thus, investigations regarding prescribed exercise following bariatric weight loss surgery are scarce.

Shah et al. (2011) randomized individuals at least three months post-surgery into a high volume exercise program (HVEP) or control group. The HVEP consisted of 12 weeks of aerobic exercise at 60-70% of VO_{2max} with a weekly goal of ≥2,000 kcal/week expenditure. Despite significant increased total energy expenditure ($kcal \cdot kg^{-1} \cdot day^{-1}$), HVEP did not show significantly altered outcomes for cardiorespiratory fitness, changes in LBM, reductions in fat mass, or reductions in BMI as compared to the non-exercising controls [48]. Interestingly, individuals in the HVEP did have a beneficial change in post-prandial blood glucose response to an oral glucose tolerance test [48]. Castello et al. (2011) also studied the effects of prescribed aerobic training at four months post-surgery. Individuals exercised for 12 weeks at 50-70% of peak heart rate 3 $d \cdot wk^{-1}$ for 1 $h \cdot day^{-1}$ [58]. The aerobic training group saw similar reductions in weight loss and reductions in BMI but significant increase in the 6MWT as compared to the non-exercising control group [58]. A combination of resistance training (2 sets, 15 reps, 60-75% 1-RM) and aerobic training (30 $min \cdot d^{-1}$, 60-75% heart rate reserve; HHR: defined as difference between resting heart rate and peak heart rate) was completed 3 $d \cdot wk^{-1}$ for 12 weeks in surgery patients in the study by Stegan et al. (2011). Both the training group and non-exercising controls saw similar improvements in body weight, BMI, and aerobic capacity [59]. However, the combination training prevented reductions in muscle strength of major muscle groups as compared to non-exercising controls [59].

Together these studies do not show significant enhancements of surgical outcomes (excess weight loss and BMI reductions) with the addition of a post-operative exercise regimen. This may be due to the large reductions in weight already associated with weight loss surgery, which may confound each study's ability to identify significant differences. Furthermore, these studies follow these individuals for only 12 weeks, in which the time frame may not be long enough to identify the long-term benefits of exercise interventions in these populations. However, enhancements in glucose tolerance [48] and maintenance of muscle mass [59] was seen within these time frames, indicating positive health benefits.

Optimization of Exercise Strategies Following Surgery

Until exercise specialists have more data concerning the effects of weight loss surgery on fitness and physical activity patterns, it is difficult to effectively prescribe exercise plans during the post-surgical period, either acutely or over the long-term. In general, addition of overall PA via increased aerobic exercise should facilitate fat loss while maintaining lean mass. Sufficient doses of aerobic exercise should also improve cardiorespiratory and cardiometabolic fitness. Accentuation of this prescription with some resistance training may ameliorate the losses in muscle mass seen in some post-bariatric surgery patients.

Current American College of Sports Medicine recommendations suggest 30 min·d^{-1} on 5 d·wk^{-1} at a moderate to vigorous (60-75% maximal capacity) for enhancements of cardiorespiratory fitness [3, 14]. Maximal capacity may be determined in a variety of ways such as the VO_{2max}, maximal predicted heart rate (HR_{max}; HR_{max} = 220 – Age), or the heart rate reserve (HRR; HRR= Maximal heart rate – resting heart rate). However, evidence suggests that 150 min·wk^{-1} of moderate to vigorous physical activity is effective at preventing weight gain, while additional amounts of time (~250 min·wk^{-1}) can result in modest weight loss [60]. Exercise amounts greater 250 min· wk^{-1} may be required for prevention of weight regain in the previously overweight [60]. Until more controlled randomized trails regarding various exercise interventions exploring the amounts, durations, intensities, and modalities of exercise strategies are available, further recommendations for cannot be prescribed.

Until more precise studies are done in severely obese populations, a general recommendation would be the addition of 1-3 sets of resistance exercise to the aerobic exercise described above. This would consist of 8-12 repetitions at 70-85% of 1-RM performed 2-3 d·wk^{-1} in all major muscle groups [17]. The goal of these exercises should be prevention of decrements in muscle strength and muscle mass that are prevalent following weight loss surgery.

Considerations for Future Investigations

We have highlighted two general areas in which further studies are needed using well-controlled designs and objective measures. The first of these is the assessment of overall physical fitness. More studies are needed using techniques such as graded exercise testing to identify the individual and interactive effects of surgery and weight loss on various aspects of overall fitness such as cardiorespiratory fitness. In addition, there is considerable interest in the loss of lean body mass in certain patients following weight loss surgery, such that body composition longitudinal assessments are warranted, rather than relying on BMI (which does not speak to composition) to indicate morphologic changes. Fitness changes in patients are likely also modified by a litany of factors, including gender, age, and race, as well as baseline levels for fitness and history of physical activities. The second area we highlighted as needing more study is changes in physical activity levels after surgery-induced weight loss. While we reviewed a number of studies in the literature concerning physical activity in post-surgical patients, there is a severe lack of both objectively-measured general physical activity levels and purposeful prescribed exercise intervention studies to see how exercise affects tissues in the time period after weight loss surgery. Together, these data can be integrated to provide more precise exercise prescriptions post-surgery to facilitate health improvements.

References

[1] Buchwald H, Oien DM. Metabolic/bariatric surgery worldwide 2011. *Obesity Surgery.* 2013;23(4):427-36.

[2] Blair SN, Kohl HW, 3rd, Barlow CE, Paffenbarger RS, Jr., Gibbons LW, Macera CA. Changes in physical fitness and all-cause mortality. A prospective study of healthy and unhealthy men. *JAMA.* 1995;273(14):1093-8.

[3] American College of Sports Medicine Position Stand. Quantity and quality of exercise for developing and maintaining cardiorespiratory, musculoskeletal, and neuromotor fitness in apparently healthy adults: guidance for prescribing exercise. *Medicine and science in sports and exercise.* 2011;43(7):1334-59.

[4] Physical Activity Guidelines Advisory Committee report, 2008. To the Secretary of Health and Human Services. Part A: executive summary. *Nutrition reviews.* 2009;67(2):114-20.

[5] Kolotkin RL, LaMonte MJ, Litwin S, Crosby RD, Gress RE, Yanowitz FG, et al. Cardiorespiratory fitness and health-related quality of life in bariatric surgery patients. *Obesity surgery.* 2011;21(4):457-64.

[6] de Souza SA, Faintuch J, Sant'anna AF. Effect of weight loss on aerobic capacity in patients with severe obesity before and after bariatric surgery. *Obesity Surgery.* 2010;20(7):871-5.

[7] Kolotkin RL, Head S, Hamilton M, Tse CK. Assessing Impact of Weight on Quality of Life. *Obesity Research.* 1995;3(1):49-56.

[8] Buchwald H, Avidor Y, Braunwald E, Jensen MD, Pories W, Fahrbach K, et al. Bariatric surgery: a systematic review and meta-analysis. *JAMA.* 2004;292(14):1724-37.

[9] Magro DO, Geloneze B, Delfini R, Pareja BC, Callejas F, Pareja JC. Long-term weight regain after gastric bypass: a 5-year prospective study. *Obesity surgery.* 2008;18(6):648-51.

[10] Freire RH, Borges MC, Alvarez-Leite JI, Toulson Davisson Correia MI. Food quality, physical activity, and nutritional follow-up as determinant of weight regain after Roux-en-Y gastric bypass. *Nutrition.* 2012;28(1):53-8.

[11] Faria SL, de Oliveira Kelly E, Lins RD, Faria OP. Nutritional management of weight regain after bariatric surgery. *Obesity surgery.* 2010;20(2):135-9.

[12] Caspersen CJ, Powell KE, Christenson GM. Physical activity, exercise, and physical fitness: definitions and distinctions for health-related research. *Public health reports.* 1985;100(2):126-31.

[13] Corbin CB, Pangrazi, R.P., Franks, D.B.,. Definitions: Health, Fitness, and Physical Activity. *Research Digest.* 2000:11.

[14] Pescatello LS, American College of Sports Medicine. *ACSM's guidelines for exercise testing and prescription.* 9th ed. Philadelphia: Wolters Kluwer/Lippincott Williams & Wilkins Health; 2014. xxiv, 456 p. p.

[15] Haskell WL, Lee IM, Pate RR, Powell KE, Blair SN, Franklin BA, et al. Physical activity and public health: updated recommendation for adults from the American College of Sports Medicine and the American Heart Association. *Medicine and Science in Sports and Exercise.* 2007;39(8):1423-34.

[16] Goodpaster BH, Delany JP, Otto AD, Kuller L, Vockley J, South-Paul JE, et al. Effects of diet and physical activity interventions on weight loss and cardiometabolic risk factors in severely obese adults: a randomized trial. *JAMA.* 2010;304(16):1795-802.

[17] American College of Sports M. American College of Sports Medicine Position Stand. Progression models in resistance training for healthy adults. *Medicine and Science in Sports and Exercise.* 2009;41(3):687-708.

[18] Selye H. Stress and the general adaptation syndrome. *British Medical Journal.* 1950;1(4667):1383-92.

[19] Nelson ME, Rejeski WJ, Blair SN, Duncan PW, Judge JO, King AC, et al. Physical activity and public health in older adults: recommendation from the American College of Sports Medicine and the American Heart Association. *Circulation.* 2007;116(9):1094-105.

[20] United States. Department of Health and Human Services. *2008 physical activity guidelines for Americans: be active, healthy, and happy!* Washington, DC: U.S. Dept. of Health and Human Services; 2008. ix, 61 p. p.

[21] Brooks GA, Fahey TD, Baldwin KM. *Exercise physiology: human bioenergetics and its applications.* 4th ed. Boston: McGraw-Hill; 2005. xxi, 876, 7, 22 p. p.

[22] Roche AF, Heymsfield S, Lohman TG. *Human body composition.* Champaign, IL: Human Kinetics; 1996. x, 366 p. p.

[23] Pollack ML, Schmidt DH, Jackson AS. Measurement of cardio-respiratory fitness and body composition in the clinical setting. *Comprehensive Therapy.* 1980;6(9):12-27.

[24] Rimm EB, Stampfer MJ, Giovannucci E, Ascherio A, Spiegelman D, Colditz GA, et al. Body size and fat distribution as predictors of coronary heart disease among middle-aged and older US men. *American Journal of Epidemiology.* 1995;141(12):1117-27.

[25] Alexander JK. Obesity and Cardiac Performance. *The American Journal of Cardiology.* 1964;14:860-5.

[26] Barlow CE, Kohl HW, 3rd, Gibbons LW, Blair SN. Physical fitness, mortality and obesity. *International journal of obesity and related metabolic disorders: Journal of the International Association for the Study of Obesity.* 1995;19 Suppl 4:S41-4.

[27] Ekelund LG, Haskell WL, Johnson JL, Whaley FS, Criqui MH, Sheps DS. Physical fitness as a predictor of cardiovascular mortality in asymptomatic North American men. The Lipid Research Clinics Mortality Follow-up Study. *The New England Journal of Medicine.* 1988;319(21):1379-84.

[28] Laukkanen JA, Lakka TA, Rauramaa R, Kuhanen R, Venalainen JM, Salonen R, et al. Cardiovascular fitness as a predictor of mortality in men. *Archives of Internal Medicine.* 2001;161(6):825-31.

[29] Salvadori A, Fanari P, Fontana M, Buontempi L, Saezza A, Baudo S, et al. Oxygen uptake and cardiac performance in obese and normal subjects during exercise. *Respiratio.* 1999;66(1):25-33.

[30] Sandvik L, Erikssen J, Thaulow E, Erikssen G, Mundal R, Rodahl K. Physical fitness as a predictor of mortality among healthy, middle-aged Norwegian men. *The New England Journal of Medicine.* 1993;328(8):533-7.

[31] Wei M, Kampert JB, Barlow CE, Nichaman MZ, Gibbons LW, Paffenbarger RS, Jr., et al. Relationship between low cardiorespiratory fitness and mortality in normal-weight, overweight, and obese men. *JAMA.* 1999;282(16):1547-53.

[32] McCullough PA, Gallagher MJ, Dejong AT, Sandberg KR, Trivax JE, Alexander D, et al. Cardiorespiratory fitness and short-term complications after bariatric surgery. *Chest.* 2006;130(2):517-25.

[33] Chaston TB, Dixon JB, O'Brien PE. Changes in fat-free mass during significant weight loss: a systematic review. *International Journal of Obesity.* 2007;31(5):743-50.

[34] Tamboli RA, Hossain HA, Marks PA, Eckhauser AW, Rathmacher JA, Phillips SE, et al. Body composition and energy metabolism following Roux-en-Y gastric bypass surgery. *Obesity.* 2010;18(9):1718-24.

[35] Leite FS, Barbalho-Moulim MC, Soares KK, Dias F, D., Peixoto-Souza FS, Costa D. Evaluation of functional capacity, body composition and pulmonary function after bariatric surgery. *Health.* 2013;5(8A3):7.

[36] Vargas CB, Picolli F, Dani C, Padoin AV, Mottin CC. Functioning of obese individuals in pre- and postoperative periods of bariatric surgery. *Obesity Surgery.* 2013;23(10):1590-5.

[37] Barbalho-Moulim MC, Miguel GP, Forti EM, Campos Fdo A, Peixoto-Souza FS, Costa D. Pulmonary Function after Weight Loss in Obese Women Undergoing Roux-en-Y Gastric Bypass: One-Year Followup. *ISRN Obesity.* 2013;2013:796454.

[38] Bond DS, Jakicic JM, Unick JL, Vithiananthan S, Pohl D, Roye GD, et al. Pre- to postoperative physical activity changes in bariatric surgery patients: self report vs. objective measures. *Obesity.* 2010;18(12):2395-7.

[39] Boan J, Kolotkin RL, Westman EC, McMahon RL, Grant JP. Binge eating, quality of life and physical activity improve after Roux-en-Y gastric bypass for morbid obesity. *Obesity Surgery.* 2004;14(3):341-8.

[40] Bond DS, Evans RK, Wolfe LG, Meador JG, Sugerman HJ, Kellum JM, et al. Impact of self-reported physical activity participation on proportion of excess weight loss and BMI among gastric bypass surgery patients. *The American Surgeon.* 2004;70(9):811-4.

[41] Silver HJ, Torquati A, Jensen GL, Richards WO. Weight, dietary and physical activity behaviors two years after gastric bypass. *Obesity Surgery.* 2006;16(7):859-64.

[42] Mathus-Vliegen EM, de Wit LT. Health-related quality of life after gastric banding. *The British Journal of Surgery.* 2007;94(4):457-65.

[43] Welch G, Wesolowski C, Piepul B, Kuhn J, Romanelli J, Garb J. Physical activity predicts weight loss following gastric bypass surgery: findings from a support group survey. *Obesity Surgery.* 2008;18(5):517-24.

[44] Colles SL, Dixon JB, O'Brien PE. Hunger control and regular physical activity facilitate weight loss after laparoscopic adjustable gastric banding. *Obesity Surgery.* 2008;18(7):833-40.

[45] Bond DS, Phelan S, Wolfe LG, Evans RK, Meador JG, Kellum JM, et al. Becoming physically active after bariatric surgery is associated with improved weight loss and health-related quality of life. *Obesity.* 2009;17(1):78-83.

[46] Livhits M, Mercado C, Yermilov I, Parikh JA, Dutson E, Mehran A, et al. Behavioral factors associated with successful weight loss after gastric bypass. *The American Surgeon.* 2010;76(10):1139-42.

[47] Forbush S, Nof L, Echternach J, Hill C, Rainey J. Influence of activity levels and energy intake on percent excess weight loss after Roux-en-Y gastric bypass. *Obesity Surgery.* 2011;21(11):1731-8.

[48] Shah M, Snell PG, Rao S, Adams-Huet B, Quittner C, Livingston EH, et al. High-volume exercise program in obese bariatric surgery patients: a randomized, controlled trial. *Obesity.* 2011;19(9):1826-34.

[49] Josbeno DA, Kalarchian M, Sparto PJ, Otto AD, Jakicic JM. Physical activity and physical function in individuals post-bariatric surgery. *Obesity Surgery.* 2011;21(8):1243-9.

[50] Vatier C, Henegar C, Ciangura C, Poitou-Bernert C, Bouillot JL, Basdevant A, et al. Dynamic relations between sedentary behavior, physical activity, and body composition after bariatric surgery. *Obesity Surgery.* 2012;22(8):1251-6.

[51] Mundi MS, Lorentz PA, Swain J, Grothe K, Collazo-Clavell M. Moderate physical activity as predictor of weight loss after bariatric surgery. *Obesity Surgery.* 2013;23(10):1645-9.

[52] Egberts K, Brown WA, Brennan L, O'Brien PE. Does exercise improve weight loss after bariatric surgery? A systematic review. *Obesity Surgery.* 2012;22(2):335-41.

[53] Evans RK, Bond DS, Wolfe LG, Meador JG, Herrick JE, Kellum JM, et al. Participation in 150 min/wk of moderate or higher intensity physical activity yields greater weight loss after gastric bypass surgery. *Surgery for Obesity and Related Diseases.* 2007;3(5):526-30.

[54] Chevallier JM, Paita M, Rodde-Dunet MH, Marty M, Nogues F, Slim K, et al. Predictive factors of outcome after gastric banding: a nationwide survey on the role of center activity and patients' behavior. *Annals of Surgery.* 2007;246(6):1034-9.

[55] Anderson JW, Brinkman VL, Hamilton CC. Weight loss and 2-y follow-up for 80 morbidly obese patients treated with intensive very-low-calorie diet and an education program. *The American Journal of Clinical Nutrition.* 1992;56(1 Suppl):244S-6S.

[56] Ryan DH, Johnson WD, Myers VH, Prather TL, McGlone MM, Rood J, et al. Nonsurgical weight loss for extreme obesity in primary care settings: results of the Louisiana Obese Subjects Study. *Archives of Internal Medicine.* 2010;170(2):146-54.

[57] Samaha FF, Iqbal N, Seshadri P, Chicano KL, Daily DA, McGrory J, et al. A low-carbohydrate as compared with a low-fat diet in severe obesity. *The New England Journal of Medicine.* 2003;348(21):2074-81.

[58] Castello V, Simoes RP, Bassi D, Catai AM, Arena R, Borghi-Silva A. Impact of aerobic exercise training on heart rate variability and functional capacity in obese women after gastric bypass surgery. *Obesity Surgery.* 2011;21(11):1739-49.

[59] Stegen S, Derave W, Calders P, Van Laethem C, Pattyn P. Physical fitness in morbidly obese patients: effect of gastric bypass surgery and exercise training. *Obesity surgery.* 2011;21(1):61-70.

[60] American College of Sports Medicine Position Stand. Appropriate physical activity intervention strategies for weight loss and prevention of weight regain for adults. *Medicine and Science In Sports and Exercise.* 2009;41(2):459-71.

In: Bariatric Surgery
Editor: Mandy Chambers

ISBN: 978-1-63463-697-1

Chapter 2

Small Intestinal Bacterial Overgrowth after Bariatric Surgery

Iman Andalib, MD,[1] Naveen Gara, MD,[1] Bikram S. Bal, MD[2], Timothy R. Shope, MD,[3] and Timothy R. Koch, MD[1,*]

[1]Section of Gastroenterology and Hepatology, Washington, DC, US
[2]Center for Gastrointestinal and Liver Diseases, Centra Southside, Farmville, VA, US
[3]Department of Surgery, MedStar-Washington Hospital Center and Georgetown University School of Medicine, Washington, DC, US

Abstract

Worldwide, the prevalence of obesity continues to rise. Attempts at modification of diet and lifestyle often fail to prevent the medical complications of obesity. Bariatric surgery is being increasingly utilized for treatment of obesity. Despite being a gold standard therapy for management of medically-complicated obesity, bariatric surgery has been associated with multiple complications including nutritional deficiencies, bloating, and dyspepsia. Ongoing clinical research has shown that bariatric surgery can lead to postoperative small intestinal bacterial overgrowth with its related nutritional deficiencies. Bacterial overgrowth may result from alteration of the host defense mechanisms, including loss of gastric acid or diminished exposure to bile acids, and altered upper gastrointestinal motility. Other co-morbid disorders, including diabetes mellitus, chronic narcotic use, use of proton pump inhibitors and antidepressants appear to play a role in the development of bacterial overgrowth. Although microbial investigation of jejunal aspirates is the gold standard for detecting bacterial overgrowth, glucose-hydrogen breath testing is increasingly becoming the test of choice for this diagnosis. The treatment for bacterial overgrowth can be very challenging and can include treatment of the underlying disease, correction of vitamin deficiencies, and

* Correspondence to: Timothy R. Koch, M.D., Professor of Medicine (Gastroenterology), Georgetown University School of Medicine, Center for Advanced Laparoscopic & Bariatric Surgery, POB North, Suite 3400, MedStar-Washington Hospital Center, 110 Irving Street, NW, Washington, DC 20010 United States. Email: timothy.r.koch@medstar.net. Telephone and fax: Telephone: +1-202 8777788; FAX: +1-877 6808198.

discontinuation of motility-altering medications. Antibiotics are effective, but only a few studies concerning choice of and duration of antibiotic therapy exist. Herein, we describe the potential mechanisms for the development of small intestinal bacterial overgrowth, the effects of bacterial overgrowth on nutrients, the methods of diagnosis of bacterial overgrowth, and treatment options for this disorder.

Introduction

Microbiota of the Alimentary Tract

Small intestinal bacterial overgrowth (SIBO) results in a malabsorption syndrome due to an increase in and/or alteration of microorganisms within the upper gastrointestinal tract. It is a condition in which there is an expansion of bacteria in the small intestine resulting in excessive fermentation and malabsorption, which can significantly impair an individual's quality of life.

This is not a new surgical disorder. In a 1955 publication, Dr. James Halsted commented that: "intestinal anastomosis leading to stasis of intestinal contents, with overgrowth of bacteria, may cause vitamin B12 deficiency through bacterial interference" [1]. Early work demonstrated that concentrations of the bacterial flora in the gastrointestinal tract normally vary along the length of the gastrointestinal tract [2].

In human physiology, bacterial fermentation is limited to the distal gut as well as to the large intestine. The duodenum and jejunum are relatively sterile. Therefore, colonization of bacteria in the upper gut is abnormal. In this syndrome of SIBO, the flora of the proximal small intestine begin to resemble the flora of a healthy subject's colon, developing high concentrations of anaerobic bacteria. In patients who have undergone bariatric surgery, it would be reasonable to expect that the altered upper gut flora would resemble species present in mouth flora since individuals are frequently swallowing fluids (including saliva). This assumption however has not been confirmed by studies involving subjects after bariatric surgery.

Bacterial concentrations in the upper small intestine typically are low due to effects of gastric acid, gastric emptying, and normal small intestinal motility. The concentration of bacteria in the cecum is usually 10^{10-12} colony forming unit (cfu)/ml; in the ileum bacterial concentrations drop to 10^{5-8} cfu/ml, and in the jejunum and the duodenum bacterial concentrations further drop to 10^{0-4} cfu/ml [3-5]. Therefore, for fermentation to occur, food must normally reach the distal gut anaerobic bacteria. Expansion of bacterial populations in the upper gut can be blocked by several defense mechanisms, including the intestinal immune system, gastric acid, gastric emptying, pancreatic enzymes, intraluminal bile, and small intestinal motility (see Table 1). If any of these mechanisms fail, SIBO could then develop [6]. In addition, in the small intestine, the cleansing action of peristalsis especially the interdigestive migrating motor complex (termed MMCs) is important for the propulsion of bacteria into the colon [7]. Therefore, conditions that result in dysmotility of the small intestine could lead to upper gut bacterial overgrowth.

Table 1. Defense Factors Preventing Small Intestinal Bacterial Overgrowth

Intestinal Immune System
Gastric Acid Production
Gastric Emptying
Pancreatic Enzymes
Intraluminal Bile
Small Intestinal Motility
-Interdigestive Migrating Motor Complexes
-Small Intestinal Liquid and Solid Transit

Predisposing Factors

The etiologies of SIBO are complex and are summarized in Table 2. The origin of SIBO includes clinical disorders and anatomical abnormalities such as bariatric surgery, partial gastrectomy with Billroth II reconstruction, small intestinal diverticulosis, small intestinal stricture (due to Crohn's disease, radiation enteritis, or focal segmental ischemia), fistulae, or previous resection of the ileo-cecal valve. Other predisposing factors involve disorders of protective antibacterial mechanisms including the presence of pancreatic insufficiency or achlorhydria [7]. Motility disorders that can induce SIBO include scleroderma, diabetes mellitus with autonomic neuropathy, or chronic idiopathic intestinal pseudo-obstruction. Other disorders associated with SIBO include celiac disease, chronic pancreatitis, and radiation enteritis [7-9].

Table 2. Clinical Conditions and the Development of Small Intestinal Bacterial Overgrowth

Anatomical Alteration
Bariatric Surgery
Small Intestinal Diverticulosis
Intestinal Stricture (Benign, Malignant, Radiation-Induced or Crohn's disease)
Fistula (Gastrocolic or Jejunocolic; Crohn's disease)
Resection of Ileocecal Valve
Altered Gastric Acid Production
Post-Surgical Gastrectomy or Vagotomy
Chronic *Helicobacter pylori* gastritis
Proton Pump Inhibitor
Dysmotility Disorders
Gut Autonomic Neuropathy (Diabetes Mellitus)
Scleroderma
Motility-Altering Medications (Narcotics, Anti-Depressants, or Calcium-Channel Antagonists)
Medical Disorders
Immunodeficiency Disorders
Celiac Disease
Chronic Pancreatitis

There are reports in the literature that use of chronic narcotics, proton pump inhibitors, and antidepressants could increase the likelihood of developing SIBO, but these factors have not been extensively studied [10].

We have evaluated the association between medication use and SIBO in patients after Roux-en-Y gastric bypass [11]. In a retrospective study that included 206 patients who underwent Roux-en-Y gastric bypass at our institution from 1999-2007, all patients were required to take a daily multivitamin with minerals. A serum folate level above the upper limit of normal was considered to be elevated and therefore consistent with a diagnosis of SIBO [12-13]. There were 115 patients (97 females and 18 males; average age: 46 years-old; average BMI: 53 kg/m^2) who had serum folate levels measured. Medication lists for these patients after gastric bypass were reviewed, and short-term narcotic use in the immediate post-operative period was excluded. There were 58 patients with chronic narcotic use of whom 51 had elevated serum folate levels; in a control group of 32 patients who received no motility-altering medication, only 10 patients had elevated serum folate levels (Chi-squared 2x2: $p<.0001$). This result supported the strong relationship between chronic narcotic usage and SIBO. Among the 25 remaining patients, 13 of 13 patients (100%) who were receiving an anti-depressant medication had elevated serum folate levels, 8 of 9 patients (89%) who were receiving a proton pump inhibitor had elevated serum folate levels, and 2 of 3 patients (67%) who were receiving a calcium channel antagonist had elevated serum folate levels. These results support the concern that patients after bariatric surgery may be at risk for development of SIBO during concomitant intake of narcotics, proton pump inhibitors, anti-depressants, or calcium-channel antagonists.

SIBO has been identified by clinical evidence and abnormal glucose-breath tests in patients who have undergone Roux-en-Y gastric bypass (as discussed above), vertical sleeve gastrectomy, and adjustable gastric banding.

It has been suggested that inadequate small intestinal motility may result in the presence of residual food particles or residue in the small intestine, a potential culture media for bacteria. Specifically, a reduction in the frequency or occurrence of interdigestive (fasting) migrating motor complexes (MMC) could result in the development of small bowel bacterial overgrowth. However, a study from the Mayo Clinic (Rochester, MN) reported however significant increases in the frequency of phase III MMCs in individuals who had undergone partial gastrectomy with either Billroth II reconstruction or Roux-en-Y reconstruction [14].

By contrast, investigators at the University of Copenhagen (Denmark) studied 17 individuals after Roux-en-Y gastric bypass and compared their results to 9 controls [15]. Small intestinal transit was examined using gamma camera images in individuals receiving mixed isotope solid-liquid meals. The passage of solid isotope, but not liquid isotope, was significantly prolonged through the small intestine in individuals who had undergone Roux-en-Y gastric bypass. Slowed passage of solids through the small intestine could be an important factor promoting the overgrowth of upper gut bacteria.

Advanced age may be an independent risk factor for SIBO [16]. However, the incidence of SIBO may be underestimated, since many of these patients are asymptomatic. The underlying mechanism has been proposed to be due to age-related dysmotility or achlorhydria (possibly caused by atrophic gastritis induced by chronic gastric *Helicobacter pylori* infection). Further studies are needed to determine the actual incidence of SIBO in this population.

Mechanisms of Malabsorption

Proposed mechanisms of malabsorption in individuals with SIBO are summarized in Table 3. Bacteria in the small intestine can interrupt the metabolism and absorption of many bioactive compounds including monosaccharides, lipids, proteins and vitamins [1, 13, 17, 18].

Table 3. Proposed Mechanisms of Malabsorption Induced by Small Intestinal Bacterial Overgrowth

Bacterial Deconjugation of Bile Salts
Reduced Brush Border Disaccharidases
Carbohydrate Fermentation by Bacteria
Formation of Short-Chain Organic Acids
Utilization of Protein by Bacteria
Altered Gut Permeability
Utilization of Vitamins by Bacteria
Interference with the Cobalamin-Intrinsic Factor Complex

Fat malabsorption in SIBO has been proposed to result from bacterial deconjugation of bile salts in the proximal gut. Conjugated bile salts are required for micelle formation (containing lipids and fat-soluble vitamins A, D, E and K) prior to micelle absorption in the terminal ileum. However, in individuals with SIBO, bacteria in the small intestine deconjugate bile salts forming free bile acids, which can interfere with formation of mixed micelles. Furthermore, deconjugated bile acids formed by bacterial activity may induce mucosal damage, and thus contribute to patchy submucosal lesions identified in individuals with SIBO.

Although malabsorption of lipophilic vitamins (vitamins A, D, E, and K) may also occur as a result of altered micelle absorption, vitamin K levels are generally normal in patients with SIBO due to the production of vitamin K by luminal bacteria [17-19].

Carbohydrate malabsorption is also common in SIBO. This phenomenon has been proposed to be the result of reduced brush border disaccharidase levels (due to digestion by bacterial proteases) as well as carbohydrate fermentation by the bacteria, itself. In addition, small intestinal and colonic bacteria can metabolize these malabsorbed carbohydrates to form short-chain organic acids, which leads to increased osmolarity of the intestinal fluid and thus results in diarrhea [17, 20].

Protein malabsorption has been proposed to be the consequence of utilization of protein by the bacteria. Another proposed mechanism may be the enterocyte injury which alters the gut permeability leading to the development of a protein-losing enteropathy [21].

The postoperative development of vitamin B12 deficiency induced by SIBO has a complex pathophysiology. In a healthy proximal small intestine, intrinsic factor normally binds to vitamin B12. This complex will facilitate cobalamin absorption in the distal ileum. In the presence of SIBO, the colonized bacteria including anaerobes and facultative gram-negative aerobes utilize or consume vitamin B12 making it less available for absorption. In SIBO, bacteria can interfere with the formation of the cobalamin-intrinsic factor complex.

Interestingly, enteric bacteria do biosynthesize cobalamin. However, this cobalamin is not available for absorption by the host as it is retained by the bacteria [3, 17, 22].

Effects of Small Intestinal Bacterial Overgrowth on Nutrition

Small intestinal bacterial overgrowth may include a catabolic process that could lower serum albumin levels. The preoperative prevalence of hypoalbuminemia in patients seeking bariatric surgery is reported to be 1.1% [23]. Clinicians in Brazil have reported two patients who developed hypoalbuminemia after Roux-en-Y gastric bypass [24]. Hydrogen breath testing supported a diagnosis of bacterial overgrowth. Each patient was treated with oral ciprofloxacin for two weeks and one patient in addition received a two week course of oral tetracycline. One patient had a rise in serum albumin from 2.4 g/dl pre-treatment to 3.3 g/dl post-treatment, while in the second patient, the serum albumin pre-treatment was 2.3 g/dl but the post-treatment level was only 2.7 g/dl (normal range is 3.5 to 5.0 g/dl).

Upon examination of patients who underwent Roux-en-Y gastric bypass surgery at our institution from 1999-2007, we identified 115 individuals who had both serum folate and serum albumin levels obtained [25]. A serum folate level above the upper limit of normal was considered to be an indirect measure of small intestinal bacterial overgrowth [12, 13], and a serum albumin level below the lower limit of normal was considered to be low. In this study, 42 patients with an abnormal glucose-hydrogen breath test, consistent with SIBO, were treated with oral antibiotics. There was no relationship identified between SIBO and low serum albumin levels (Chi-squared 2x2: p=0.8). Among 42 patients with abnormal glucose-hydrogen breath test, 14 patients (33%) had low serum albumin levels and 42% of these patients achieved normal serum albumin levels after antibiotic treatment for SIBO (see Figure 1). Thus, there was no evidence that SIBO induced hypoalbuminemia; treatment of SIBO did not improve serum albumin levels in the majority of patients after Roux-en-Y gastric bypass.

In an attempt to suppress the development of SIBO, Woodard and associates followed 44 patients after Roux-en-Y gastric bypass who were randomized to receive either a control (placebo) or 2.4 billion Lactobacillus species daily [26]. At 6 months, individuals who received daily Lactobacillus had reduced breath hydrogen levels, supporting suppression of upper gut bacterial overgrowth. However, there were no differences in weight loss when comparing the two groups of patients at 6 months. It was noted that gastrointestinal quality of life surveys had improved in both groups, supporting the importance of gastric bypass surgery in improving patients' quality of life.

In examination of the effect of SIBO on vitamin B12, SIBO classically causes megaloblastic anemia [1]. Cobalamin (vitamin B12) deficiency can occur as a result of utilization of the vitamin by the bacteria before it can be absorbed. This deficiency is improved after antibiotic administration, but cannot be corrected by addition of intrinsic factor.

We have reported the effect of SIBO on vitamin B1 (thiamine) levels after Roux-en-Y gastric bypass [13]. There was a significant relationship between the presence of SIBO and whole blood thiamine diphosphate levels that were below the lower limit of normal.

Twenty one patients were also evaluated who had thiamine diphosphate levels below the lower limit of normal and abnormal glucose-hydrogen breath tests, consistent with SIBO [13]. Fifteen patients received oral thiamine supplements, but repeat whole blood thiamine levels remained low in all 15. Nine of these patients then received oral antibiotic therapy. Determination of repeat thiamine levels revealed that all 9 patients had normalized their whole blood thiamine levels. These results support the hypothesis that SIBO induces thiamine deficiency after gastric bypass surgery in obese patients. Patients after gastric bypass surgery who develop thiamine deficiency may require antibiotic treatment of SIBO in order to normalize their whole blood thiamine levels.

Management

Clinical Features

As discussed above, SIBO is generally considered to be a malabsorption disorder. The clinical consequences of SIBO are similar regardless of the underlying predisposing factors (see Table 4). Patients with SIBO may be asymptomatic or may have symptoms that resemble the irritable bowel syndrome, including diarrhea, abdominal bloating, abdominal cramps, or flatulence. These symptoms are usually followed by the development of malabsorption. In patients with short bowel syndrome, inflammatory bowel diseases, scleroderma, radiation enteritis or diabetes, it may be difficult to determine whether the symptoms are due to the primary disease, or SIBO itself [3].

Many patients with SIBO fulfill Rome I criteria for a clinical diagnosis of irritable bowel syndrome, because the symptoms of SIBO and irritable bowel syndrome overlap to a large degree. Pimentel et al. [3] have reported that among 202 patients meeting Rome I criteria for IBS, 78% had abnormal breath tests, supporting the presence of SIBO. In their reports, successful eradication of SIBO after antibiotic treatment was associated with significant relief of abdominal symptoms [27]. One of the late features of SIBO is development of anemia. It is usually due to vitamin B12 deficiency, which results in macrocytic and megaloblastic anemia. In prolonged cases of malabsorption, cobalamin deficiency can lead to subacute combined degeneration of the spinal cord and/or peripheral neuropathy. In other severe cases, symptoms such as night blindness (nyctalopia) due to vitamin A deficiency, osteomalacia due to vitamin D deficiency, or vitamin E deficiency syndromes (retinopathy, anemia, ataxia, myopathy, or dysarthria) can occur. Protein malabsorption in SIBO can lead to hypoalbuminemia, which can induce peripheral edema [3].

Table 4. Clinical Features of Small Intestinal Bacterial Overgrowth

Diarrhea
Abdominal Bloating
Abdominal Cramps
Flatulence
Macrocytic Anemia
Subacute Combined Degeneration
Peripheral Neuropathy
Nyctalopia
Osteomalacia
Peripheral Edema

Diagnosis

A patient with symptoms of diarrhea, abdominal bloating/pain, or steathorrhea with a coexisting predisposition to SIBO should prompt the clinician to consider testing for small intestinal bacterial overgrowth, especially if there has been no response to empiric treatment. The "Gold Standard" for the diagnosis of a SIBO is a quantitative microbial investigation of a jejunal aspiration [6, 28]. However, this test has fallen out of favor since it has major limitations. First, in order for this quantitative test to be diagnostic, a duodenal aspirate must be obtained and then should be immediately cultured in order to identify the presence of at least 10^6 cfu/mL [29]. Second, the distribution of bacterial overgrowth might be restricted to one particular area of intestine, which may not be within the reach of a gastroscope. Since a gastroscope reaches only the upper portion of small intestine, there could be potentially high false-negative rate when using this approach for the diagnosis of SIBO [3, 30]. Since this quantitative test is invasive, time-consuming, and may be altered by contamination, breath tests such as the xylose breath test and the hydrogen breath test have been developed.

However, there is presently no general agreement as to which test is superior for the diagnosis of SIBO. ^{14}C-cholylglycine or bile acid breath test was the first encouraging breath test for the diagnosis of SIBO [31]. The test was based on the deconjugation of the bile salt by small bowel bacteria, before reaching colonic bacteria. However, it was shown that the test had a high false-negative rate of 30% to 40% with only moderate sensitivity. In addition, there was a concern of falsely positive test results in patients with ileal resection, since the unabsorbed bile salt would reach the colonic bacteria and would be deconjugated [21, 32]. With the development of newer tests, the bile acid test has fallen out of favor.

The ^{14}C-D-xylose breath test is another test with higher sensitivity and specificity. This test depends on the ability of catabolization of xylose by the high concentration of small intestine bacteria with production of $^{14}CO_2$. One of the advantages of this test is the absorption of both $^{14}CO_2$ that is produced as well as uncatabolized xylose by the proximal small bowel. These dual measurements could potentially decrease the number of false positive results caused by catabolization of xylose by colonic bacteria [7, 33]. As previously mentioned, studies have shown that the sensitivity and specificity of this test are superior to those of the ^{14}C-bile acid test [34]. Therefore, the ^{14}C-D-xylose test replaced the bile-acid breath test and became a popular test for evaluation of bacterial overgrowth. However, other investigators questioned the accuracy of this test [35], and so additional studies are needed to evaluate the efficacy of this test in patients who have undergone bariatric surgery.

Additional tests have been developed based upon the metabolic activity of upper gut bacteria. As shown in Table 5, metabolic products produced by bacteria include hydrogen, methane, ammonia, d-lactic acid and folate [13]. The pulmonary clearance of methane and hydrogen forms the pathophysiological basis for the glucose-hydrogen breath test. The glucose-hydrogen breath test has become one of the most important diagnostic methods for SIBO, with a reported sensitivity of 62.5% and a specificity of 82% [6, 28]. As shown in Figure 2 in an individual with post-prandial abdominal pain after Roux-en-Y gastric bypass, the diagnosis of a positive or abnormal glucose breath test is supported both by a high fasting breath level of methane as well as by fermentation of glucose to produce hydrogen, which is then measured in the breath.

Table 5. Metabolic Products of Bacteria

Methane
Hydrogen
Ammonia
d-Lactic Acid
Folic Acid

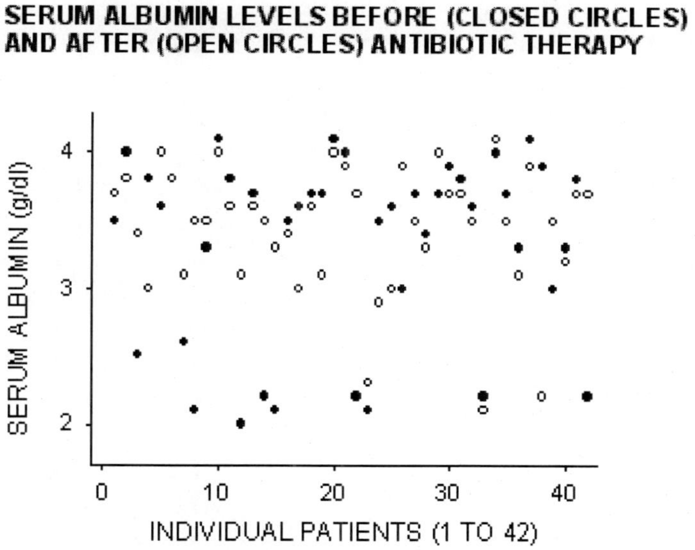

Figure 1. Effect of antibiotic therapy on serum albumin in forty two patients after Roux-en-Y gastric bypass.

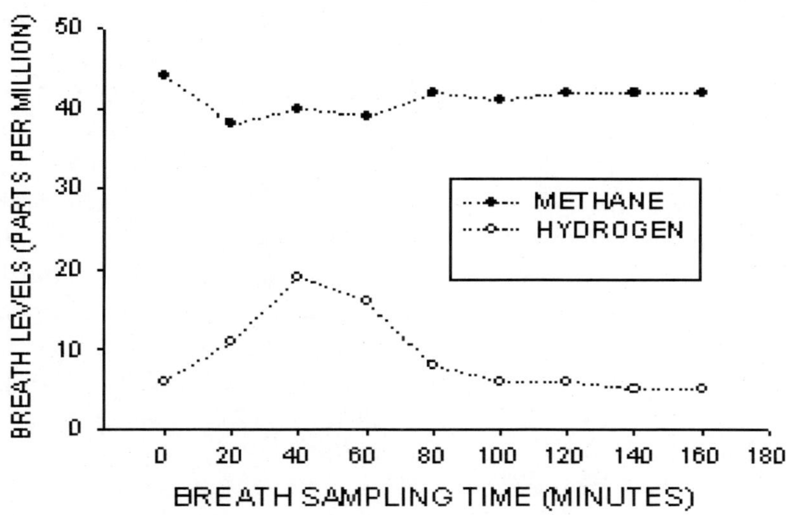

Figure 2. Gastric bypass patient with abdominal pain: breath hydrogen/methane levels after 25 grams of oral glucose.

However, there are several limitations when using the glucose-hydrogen breath test, including determination of cut-off points to define a positive test. A positive or abnormal glucose breath test in an individual who has fasted for at least 10 hours is supported by either: i. a fasting breath hydrogen or methane level that is >10 parts per million or, ii. after oral ingestion of 50 grams of glucose, an increase in breath hydrogen or methane of >14 parts per million above the baseline breath hydrogen or methane values. Furthermore, since glucose is almost completely absorbed in the proximal small intestine, this test may not be reliable for the diagnosis of SIBO of the distal small intestine. In patients with rapid transit (oral-cecal transit time of less than 75 minutes), the breath test may not be useful since it could result in false positive results [36]. As another potential downside to this test, after Roux-en-Y gastric bypass, the bypassing of duodenum and proximal jejunum could reduce absorption of glucose by the small intestine, leading to a higher percentage of patients with an abnormal breath test. Nonetheless, this test is one of the most useful methods for the diagnosis of SIBO.

Finally, the lactulose-hydrogen breath test is another test that has been examined in patients with potential SIBO, but its validity has also been questioned. In studies, it has been shown that the lactulose-hydrogen breath test has a sensitivity of 17-68% and specificity of 44-70%; therefore this test may not be useful for the diagnosis of SIBO [5].

Treatment Options

The treatment of SIBO can be complex and multifactorial. The treatment of SIBO essentially should focus on: 1) treatment of the underlying disease; 2) modification of the diet, such as a trial of a lactose-free diet; 3) discontinuation of acid-lowering or motility-altering medications; 4) correction of vitamin deficiencies and nutritional support as indicated; 5) treatment of potential dysmotility disorders; and 6) antibiotic treatment targeting the bacteria that cause SIBO.

Individuals with SIBO may be asymptomatic. However, if symptoms of malabsorption such as diarrhea and bloating occur in the presence of a positive breath test result, the clinician may decide to start antibiotic therapy for SIBO (see Table 6). There have been many studies examining different antibiotics, but no guidelines have been published with regards to the choice of antibiotics or the duration of the treatment for management of recurrent SIBO.

This is partly due to the difficulty in acquiring a culture of bacteria from the small intestine, as well as determining its antibiotic susceptibility. Generally, empiric antimicrobial agents are used that have both aerobic and anaerobic coverage. Cycling of antibiotics involves utilization of an antibiotic for 7 to 14 days, with consideration of a repeat course of antibiotic in 1 to 3 months (depending upon the timing for a return of abdominal symptoms). In addition, long-term treatment is not optimal as it might be associated with other problems such as development of antibiotic-associated diarrhea, *Clostridium difficile* colitis, and resistance to antibiotics. Also the recurrence rate of SIBO is high.

In a major meta-analysis of antibiotic treatment of SIBO, Shah and associates [37] identified 1356 articles. As their primary outcome, the authors chose normalization of post-treatment breath testing. Their secondary outcome was post-treatment clinical response. Only 10 studies met inclusion criteria. Among these 10 studies, rifaximin was studied in 8 of the studies. This meta-analysis showed that antibiotics were more effective than placebo, and that the clinical response paralleled the results obtained from breath testing.

Table 6. Antibiotic Therapy for Small Intestinal Bacterial Overgrowth

ANTIBIOTIC	DOSAGE	TIMING
Metronidazole	250-500 mg	2 to 3 Times Daily
Doxycycline	100 mg	1 to 2 Times Daily
Cefaclor	250 mg	3 Times Daily
Amoxicillin-Clavulanic Acid	250-500 mg/62.5-125 mg	2 to 3 Times Daily
Ciprofloxacin	250-500 mg	Twice Daily
Norfloxacin	400 mg	Twice Daily
Rifaximin	200-550 mg	1 to 2 Times Daily
Trimethoprim-Sulfamethoxazole	160/800 mg	1 or 2 Times Daily
Clindamycin*	150 mg	2 to 4 Times Daily

* High risk of pseudo-membranous colitis.

In older literature, the treatment of choice for SIBO was tetracycline, taken by mouth four times a day, with presumed resolution of symptoms within one week. However, new studies have shown that almost half of the patients with SIBO do not respond to this therapy, probably because tetracycline does not have a direct activity against anaerobic bacteria. Eradication rates with tetracycline were also shown to be as low as 40%.

Metronidazole has also been used for treatment of SIBO, but data are scarce with regards to this antibiotic. Metronidazole does provide coverage against anaerobic bacteria. As a potential risk factor, it has been reported that enzymatic conversion of metronidazole produces an analog of thiamine [38]. It is therefore possible that metronidazole could exacerbate thiamine deficiency induced by bacterial overgrowth in patients who have undergone bariatric surgery.

Other antibiotics such as amoxicillin–clavulanic acid have been used previously for empiric treatment of SIBO due to convenience of dosing [7]. Attar and associates compared the treatment of 10 patients with amoxicillin–clavulanic acid, norfloxacin and *Sacchromyces boulardii.* These authors identified significant improvement of symptoms with both amoxicillin–clavulanic acid (60%) and norfloxacin (90%), but no symptomatic improvement with the use of *Sacchromyces boulardii* [39].

There are additional studies which have evaluated the efficacy of non-absorbable antibiotics, including neomycin and rifaximin, to decrease the potential side effects noted with the use of systemic antibiotics. These studies have shown that rifaximin, which has bactericidal activity directed against both aerobic and anaerobic bacteria, led to the normalization of breath testing and the resolution of symptoms of malabsorption [40]. Rifaximin has also been shown to have a very low toxicity, since only < 0.4% of the drug is absorbed [41]. Neomycin has also been studied in older literature. It did not show significant clinical benefit for the treatment of SIBO, and it had no significant side effects.

Given the limited information with regards to the treatment of SIBO, there is no conclusive data to assist our understanding which antibiotics have the most efficacy. Clinicians should consider the risks of long-term systemic antibiotic therapy, costs, and the likelihood of recurrence of SIBO before choosing antibiotic treatment.

Prokinetic agents have also been evaluated due to their potential benefit for propulsion of bacteria through the small intestine. One study of 5 individuals with SIBO demonstrated a decrease in symptoms of bloating and nausea, and normalization of breath tests after nightly administration of low dose Octreotide [42]. Therefore, this agent could be an important option in those individuals who do not respond to or are intolerant to systemic antibiotics. However, this study included relatively few subjects. Additional studies are required to address questions of the effects of Octreotide, the duration of treatment with Octreotide, and whether its combination with antibiotic therapy could be beneficial to individuals with SIBO.

Although the primary goal of treatment of SIBO is to control the overgrowth of bacteria in the upper gut, nutritional support is an important component for proper management of patients with SIBO. Some of these patients have vitamin deficiencies and some patients have protein-calorie malnutrition. Therefore, appropriate nutritional supplementation with micronutrients and macronutrients is a crucial component of the treatment of SIBO.

The initial goal for treatment of protein malnutrition is the daily intake of 60 to 80 grams of protein. Multiple sources of liquid protein supplementation are commercially available. Vitamin B12 deficiency can be treated with intramuscular vitamin B12 1000 mcg once monthly. Severe vitamin B12 deficiency is treated with intramuscular vitamin B12 500-1000 mcg once daily for 7 days, then once weekly for 3 weeks, and then once monthly. In patients with control of SIBO by antibiotics, vitamin B12 deficiency may respond to oral vitamin B12 500 to 1000 mcg daily. Vitamin B1 (thiamine) deficiency can be treated with 200 mg intramuscularly once monthly. Severe thiamine deficiency (visual loss, Psychosis, or Wernicke's disease) requires 250 mg of thiamine either intramuscularly or intravenously (infusion over 3 to 4 hours) once daily for a minimum of 3 to 5 days. In patients with control of SIBO by antibiotics, vitamin B1 deficiency may respond to oral vitamin B1 100 to 250 mg twice daily.

Conclusion

Small intestinal bacterial overgrowth is a malabsorption syndrome which can lead to significant consequences such as deficiencies of macro- and micro-nutrients. It is commonly associated with other disorders and the use of acid-reducing and motility-altering medications. As the rates of bariatric surgeries rise, the risk of developing of bacterial overgrowth increases. Therefore, clinicians should always consider bacterial overgrowth in their differential as a cause of malabsorption. Due to the high incidence of bacterial overgrowth and the difficulty controlling its associated symptoms, further clinical research is warranted regarding antibiotic therapy for bacterial overgrowth. Since indefinite use of antimicrobials is not ideal therapy, further studies are needed to evaluate alternative therapies for the treatment of small intestinal bacterial overgrowth.

References

[1] Halsted, JA. Megaloblastic anemia: associated with surgically produced gastrointestinal abnormalities. *California Med* 1955; 83(3): 212-217.

[2] Finegold, SM. Intestinal bacteria: the role they play in normal physiology, pathologic physiology, and infection. *California Med* 1969; 110(6): 455-59.

[3] Lin, HC. Small intestinal bacterial overgrowth: a framework for understanding irritable bowel syndrome. *JAMA* 2004; 292(7): 852-858.

[4] Wilson, KH. The gastrointestinal biota. In: Yamada T, Alpers DH, Laine L, Owyang C, Powell DW, eds. *Textbook of Gastroenterology*. Philadelphia, PA; Williams & Wilkins; 1999; 624-636.

[5] Vanner, S. The small intestinal bacterial overgrowth irritable bowel syndrome hypothesis: implications for treatment. *Gut* 2008; 57: 1315-1321.

[6] Bures, J; Cyrany, J; Kohoutova, D; et al. Small intestinal bacterial overgrowth syndrome. *World J Gastroenterol* 2010; 16(24): 2978-2990.

[7] Singh, VV; Toskes, PP. Small bowel bacterial overgrowth: presentation, diagnosis, and treatment. *Curr Gastro Rep* 2003; 5: 365-372.

[8] Gregg, CR; Toskes, PP. Enteric bacterial flora and small bowel bacterial overgrowth syndrome. In *Sleisenger and Fordtran's Gastrointestinal and Liver Disease*, ed 7. Philadelphia, PA; WB Saunders; 2002; 1783–1793.

[9] Husebye, E; Skar, V; Hoverstad, T; et al. Abnormal intestinal motor patterns explain enteric colonization with gram-negative bacilli in late radiation enteropathy. *Gastroenterology* 1995; 109: 1078–1089.

[10] Fried, M; Siegrist, H; Frei, R; et al. Duodenal bacterial overgrowth during treatment in outpatients with omeprazole. *Gut* 1994; 35: 23–26.

[11] Bal, B; Shah, HN; Finelli, FC; Kirkpatrick, JR; Koch, TR. Risk factors associated with small intestinal bacterial overgrowth after Roux-en-Y gastric bypass surgery. *Am J Gastroenterol* 2008; 103 (S1): S97-8.

[12] Camilo, E; Zimmerman, J; Mason, JB; Golner, B; Russell, R; Selhub, J; Rosenberg, IH. Folate synthesized by bacteria in the human upper small intestine is assimilated by the host. *Gastroenterology* 1996; 110(4): 991-8.

[13] Lakhani, SV; Shah, HN; Alexander, K; Finelli, FC; Kirkpatrick, JR; Koch, TR. Small intestinal bacterial overgrowth and thiamine deficiency after Roux-en-Y gastric bypass surgery in obese patients. *Nutr Res* 2008; 28(5): 293-298.

[14] Fich, A; Neri, M; Camilleri, M; Kelly, KA; Phillips, SF. Stasis syndromes following gastric surgery: Clinical and motility features of 60 symptomatic patients. *J Clin Gastroenterol* 1990; 12(5): 505-12.

[15] Dirksen, C; Damgaard, M; Bojsen-Moller, KN; et al. Fast pouch emptying, delayed small intestinal transit, and exaggerated gut hormone responses after Roux-en-Y gastric bypass. *Neurogastroenterol Motil* 2013; 25: 346-e255.

[16] Saltzman, JR; Kowdley, KV; Pedrosa, MC; et al. Bacterial overgrowth without clinical malbsorption in elderly hypochlorhydric patients. *Gastroenterology* 1994; 106: 615–623.

[17] Koch, TR; Finelli, FC. Postoperative metabolic and nutritional complications of bariatric surgery. *Gastroenterol Clin North Am* 2010; 39(1): 109-124.

[18] Bal, B; Koch, TR; Finelli, FC; Sarr, MG. Managing medical and surgical disorders after divided Roux-en-Y gastric bypass surgery. *Nat Rev Gastroenterol Hepatol* 2010; 7: 320-324

[19] Wanitschke, R; Ammon, HV. Effects of dihydroxy bile acids and hydroxyl fatty acids on the absorption of oleic acid in the human jejunum. *J Clin Invest* 1978; 61:178–186.

[20] Giannella, RA; Rout, WR; Toskes, PP. Jejunal brush border injury and impaired sugar and amino acid uptake in the blind loop syndrome. *Gastroenterology* 1974; 67: 965–974.

[21] King, CE; Toskes, PP. Protein-losing enteropathy in the human and experimental rat blind loop syndrome. *Gastroenterology* 1981; 80: 504–509.

[22] Welkos, SA; Toskes, PP; Baer, H; et al. Importance of anaerobic bacteria in the cobalamin malabsorption of experimental rat blind loop syndrome. *Gastroenterology* 1981; 80: 313–320.

[23] Flancbaum, L; Belsley, S; Drake, V; Colarusso, T; Tayler, E. Preoperative nutritional status of patients undergoing Roux-en-Y gastric bypass for morbid obesity. *J Gastrointest Surg* 2006; 10(7): 1033-7.

[24] Machado, JDC; Campos, CS; Silva, CLD; et al. Intestinal bacterial overgrowth after Roux-en-Y gastric bypass. *Obes Surg* 2008; 18: 139-43.

[25] Bal, B; Shah, HN; Finelli, FC; Kirkpatrick, JR; Koch, TR. Hypoalbuminemia after Roux-en-Y gastric bypass surgery is not related to small intestinal bacterial overgrowth. *Am J Gastroenterol* 2008; 103 (S1): S103.

[26] Woodard, GA; Encarnacion, B; Downey, JR; et al. Probiotics improve outcomes after Roux-en-Y gastric bypass surgery: a prospective randomized trial. *J Gastrointest Surg* 2009; 13(7): 1198-204.

[27] Pimentel, M; Chow, E; Lin, HC. Eradication of small intestinal bacterial overgrowth reduces symptoms in irritable bowel syndrome. *Am J Gastroenterol* 2000; 95: 3503-3506.

[28] Gasbarrini, A; Laurittano, EC; Gabrielli, M; et al. Small intestinal bacterial overgrowth: diagnosis and treatment. *Dig Dis* 2007; 25: 237-240.

[29] Corazza, GR; Menozzi, MG; Strocchi, A; Rasciti, L; Vaira, D. The diagnosis of small bowel bacterial overgrowth: Reliability of jejunal culture and inadequacy of breath hydrogen testing. *Gastroenterology* 1990; 98: 302-309.

[30] Rumessen, JJ; Gudmand-Hoyer, E; Bachmann, E; Justesen, T. Diagnosis of bacterial overgrowth of the small intestine: comparison of the 14C-D-xylose breath test with jejunal cultures in 60 patients. *Scand J Gastroenterol* 1985; 20: 1267-1275.

[31] Fromm, H; Hofmann, AF. Breath test for altered bile acid metabolism. *Lancet* 1971; 2(7725): 621-625.

[32] Ferguson, J; Walker, K; Thomson, AB. Limitations in the use of ^{14}C-glycocholate breath and stool bile acid determinations in patients with chronic diarrhea. *J Clin Gastroenterol* 1986; 8: 258–262.

[33] King, CE; Toskes, PP. Comparison of the 1-gram [^{14}C]xylose, 10-gram lactulose-H_2, and 80-gram glucose-h_2 breath tests in patients with small intestinal bacterial overgrowth. *Gastroenterology* 1986; 91: 1447–51.

[34] Toskes, PP. The changing nature of small intestine bacterial overgrowth. Curr *Gastroenterol Rep* 1999; 1: 267–268.

[35] Lewis, SJ; Young, G; Mann, M; et al. Improvement in specificity of [^{14}C]d-xylose breath test for bacterial overgrowth. *Dig Dis Sci* 1997; 42:1587–1592.

[36] Kerlin, P; Wong, L. Breath hydrogen testing in bacterial overgrowth of the small intestine. *Gastroenterology* 1988; 95(4): 982-988.

[37] Shah, SC; Day, LW; Somsouk, M; Sewell, JL. Meta-analysis: antibiotic therapy for small intestinal bacterial overgrowth. *Aliment Pharmacol Ther* 2013; 38(8): 925-34.

[38] Alston, TA; Abeles, RH. Enzymatic conversion of the antibiotic metronidazole to an analog of thiamine. *Arch Biochem Biophys* 1987; 257(2): 357-62.

[39] Attar, A; Flourie, B; Rambaud, JC; Franchissuer, C; Ruszniewski, P; Bouhnik, Y. Antibiotic efficacy in small intestinal bacterial overgrowth-related chronic diarrhea: a crossover randomized trial. *Gastroenterology* 1999; 117: 794–797.

[40] Scrapellini, E; Gabrielli, M; Lauritano, CE; Lupascu, A; et al. High dosage rifaximin for the treatment of small intestinal bacterial overgrowth. *Aliment Pharmacol Ther* 2007; 25: 781-786.

[41] Pimentel, M; Park, S; Mirocha, J; Kane, SV; Kong, Y. The effect of a nonabsorbed oral antibiotic (rifaximin) on the symptoms of the irritable bowel syndrome. *Ann Intern Med* 2006; 145: 557-563.

[42] Soudah, HC; Hasler, WL; Owyang, C. Effect of octreotide on intestinal motility and bacterial overgrowth in scleroderma. *N Engl J Med* 1991; 325: 1461–1467.

In: Bariatric Surgery
Editor: Mandy Chambers

ISBN: 978-1-63463-697-1

Chapter 3

Complications of Bariatric Surgery, Improvement of Comorbidities and Impact on Quality of Life

Jaime Ruiz-Tovar[1]*, MD, PhD, and Carolina Llavero[2], RN
[1]Department of Surgery, General University Hospital Elche, Spain
[2]Department of Surgical Nursery, Sureste Hospital, Madrid, Spain

Abstract

More than 2/3 of the U.S, population is overweight or obese. Obesity is on the rise and the incidence is increasing most rapidly in the morbidly obese population, i.e. those with a BMIs exceeding 40 kg/m^2. Epidemiological studies estimate the prevalence of morbid obesity around 0.5%, but this rate is probably underestimated, as many morbidly obese subjects are not under any medical control. Only surgery results in substantial, long-term weight loss for obese individuals. Therefore, the performance of bariatric procedure has increased exponentially in the last 2 decades; from less than 9,000 procedures in 1993 to a high of over 115,000 in 2004. Actually, the number of bariatric procedures performed is even higher.

Despite nowadays most bariatric techniques are performed laparoscopically, the complications rate still represents a challenge for many surgeons. Complications associated to these approaches are often life-threatening conditions. Morbidly obese patients are high risk subjects and therefore, bariatric surgery must be considered a high risk procedure though the patients are operated for a benign condition. Complications include medical (deep vein thrombosis, pulmonary embolism, atelectasia, pneumonia,..) and surgical items (anastomotic leak, bleeding, surgical site infection,…).

Even considering the surgical risk, bariatric surgery has demonstrated much more advantages than disadvantages. Bariatric surgery can solve many comorbidities, such as diabetes mellitus, hypertension, dyslipidemia, pulmonary disorders, osteoarthritis,…, and reduces significantly the risk of developing new health problems, such as cardiovascular

* Correspondence to: Jaime Ruiz-Tovar, MD, PhD; Corazón de María, 64, 7° J; 28002 - Madrid (Spain); Tel: (0034)630534808; Email: jruiztovar@gmail.com.

or neoplastic events. Altogether, this leads to a significant improvement of the quality of life. The patients feel healthier and this has a positive psychological impact. There are many scales available to evaluate quality of life, but all of them coincide in that bariatric surgery achieves a significant improvement in the quality of life of morbidly obese patients.

Introduction

More than 2/3 of the U.S, population is overweight or obese. Obesity is on the rise and the incidence is increasing most rapidly in the morbidly obese population, i.e. those with BMIs exceeding 40 kg/m^2. Epidemiological studies estimate the prevalence of morbid obesity around 0.5%, but this rate is probably underestimated, as many morbidly obese subjects are not under any medical control. Only surgery results in substantial, long-term weight loss for obese individuals. Therefore, the performance of bariatric procedure has increased exponentially in the last 2 decades; from less than 9,000 procedures in 1993 to a high of over 115,000 in 2004. It is estimated that 220,000 weight-loss surgeries were performed in 2008. Actually, the number of bariatric procedures performed is even higher. [1]

Complications of Bariatric Surgery

Complications following surgical treatment of severe obesity vary based upon the procedure performed and can be as high as 40%. Due to the high surgical volume, improving the safety of these operations has become a high priority, leading to the development of strict criteria for center accreditation, guidelines for safe and effective bariatric surgery, and careful monitoring of surgical outcomes. [1, 2] Operating on obese patients is challenging because of anatomic and physiologic characteristics and comorbidities of obese patients. However, the risk of serious intra-operative and in-hospital complications and mortality rates are relatively low when the surgery is performed by experienced surgeons with an institutional investment in bariatric programs.

Postoperative complication rates vary with surgical approach, such as fewer complications with the laparoscopic approach than the open approach. Complications also vary based upon type of procedure, such as fewer complications with the adjustable gastric band (AGB) than the laparoscopic Roux-en-Y gastric bypass (LRYGB). [1-3]

Adverse Intra-Operative Events (AIE)

The adverse intra-operative event (AIE) rate varies with the complexity of the procedure, ranging in contemporary reports from <1% to 5%. [3] The most common AIE in laparoscopic surgery include:

- Anesthesia events (1%)
- Instrument/equipment failure (0.8 %)

- Bowel injury (0.8 %)
- Hepatic injury (0.4 %)
- Anastomosis revision (0.3 %)
- Splenic injury (0.2 %)
- Major blood vessel injury (0.1 %)

In addition, previous intra-abdominal operations can create extensive adhesions, and abdominal wall procedures (ie, abdominoplasty) can restrict insufflation and reduce the visible surgical field.

Trocar placement, blind insertion of the laparoscopic instruments, thermal injury or excess traction/manipulation of organs can contribute to some of the more common intra-operative laparoscopic complications.

Trocar Related Injuries

Peritoneal access by precise placement of the trocar and Veress needle is technically challenging in the patient with a thick abdominal wall; however, all types of entry access (eg, open, closed, or optical view) can be safely performed by experienced surgeons. There is no statistical difference in the rates of major complications (eg, vascular or solid organ injury) for open, closed, or optical view laparoscopic entry techniques. [4]

Spleen Injury

The spleen can be injured during weight-loss surgery, especially during a Laparoscopic sleeve gastrectomy (LSG), but bleeding can usually be controlled with hemostatic agents, and splenectomy is rarely required. [5]

Portal Vein, Inferior Vena Cava Injuries

Intra-operative injury to the portal vein and inferior vena cava is rare during bariatric operations, but can lead to rapid exsanguination. If thrombosis of the portal vein occurs following an injury, these patients require liver transplantation. [6]

Bowel Ischemia

During the performance of RYGB or BPD-DS procedures in particular, ischemia of the bowel may result if the root of the mesentery containing the mesenteric vessels is compromised or undermined during transection of the small bowel. [7]

Bowel ischemia may occur during bariatric operations in the following cases:

- Twisting the mesentery and/or mesenteric root while performing a retrocolic anastomosis for a RYGB
- Creating tension on the Roux-en-Y limb when performing a gastrojejunal anastomosis
- Incising the mesentery of the biliopancreatic limb or Roux limb at an angle such that blood flow to an end of intestinal limb is compromised.
- Closing the mesenteric defect with overly generous amounts of tissue between sutures
- Internal hernias at Petersen's defect (between the Roux limb mesentery and the transverse colon mesentery), through the transverse mesocolon itself in a retrocolic anastomosis, or the jejunojejunostomy site can also lead to ischemia and, therefore, these defects must be closed. An antecolic limb does not rule out the possibility of a future internal hernia through this potential space, but this is not likely to occur early after a RYGB.

Solid Viscus Organs

The liver can be injured during bariatric surgical procedures because of its close proximity to the stomach, especially during vertical sleeve gastrectomy. Bleeding can usually be controlled with hemostatic agents and a partial hepatectomy is rarely required. [4]

Hollow Viscus Organs

Bowel injury, such as a puncture or laceration, can occur with insertion of a Veress needle, trocar, lysis of adhesions, or dissection. [4]

Misconstruction

Misconstruction of a Roux-en-Y bypass or a biliopancreatic diversion–duodenal switch (BPD-DS) can occur during a laparoscopic or open approach. Proper bowel orientation must be maintained to avoid misconstruction. Misconstructions of the Roux-en-Y bypass with an anastomosis between the distal aspect of the biliopancreatic limb and the gastric pouch have been reported and lead to chronic bilious vomiting ("Roux-en-O"). Other examples of misconstruction include Roux limb inversion and short Roux limb. [8]

In-Hospital Postoperative Morbidity

The risk of a major complication immediately after the operation ranges from approximately 0.2% to 10% in contemporary series, depending upon patient comorbid illnesses, type of procedure, surgical approach (laparoscopic or open), and surgeon expertise.

Anastomotic Leak

The anastomotic leak remains the most dreaded technical complication of bariatric surgery and is one of the most challenging complications of weight-loss surgery. The risk of a leak ranges from 0.8% to 6%. The risk approaches 35% in revisional bariatric surgery. Most leaks occur early, generally within the first week after surgery but can occur up to a month after the operation. [9-11]

The clinical presentation is subtle and requires vigilance for signs such as low-grade fevers, respiratory compromise, and/or unexplained tachycardia greater than 120 bpm. These signs may also be present in the setting of pulmonary embolism. A leak may be radiographically confirmed by barium swallow or contrast computed tomography (CT). If a leak is suspected clinically, emergent surgical exploration should be performed, even if the imaging is negative, given the rapid progression to sepsis in the severely obese patient with comorbidities. A negative exploration that does not reveal a leak should not be considered a complication but rather evidence of good surgical judgment. Multiple studies have shown that re-exploration is safe when compared with missing or delaying the treatment of a leak. In experienced hands, surgical exploration and management of a leak is often feasible via a laparoscopic approach.

The surgical principles in treating a leak include:

- Broad-spectrum antibiotic coverage
- Identification and repair of the defect
- Irrigation and control of contamination
- Wide external drainage of the contaminated area
- Enteral access for feeding, most commonly a gastric feeding tube placed in the gastric remnant

Percutaneous drainage of a contained fluid collection may be an option in patients who are stable. Surgical therapies for persistent gastric leak are technically difficult and often unsuccessful. New approaches using minimally invasive endoscopic repair techniques appear safe and effective in some patients. These include use of glue, or placement of covered stents across the leak. Many different intraoperative techniques have been used to decrease the incidence of leaks. Over-sewing staple lines, buttressing materials for the staple line and fibrin glue have been used, but there is no evidence that these methods reliably decrease the leak rate after bypass surgery. [12,13]

Hemorrhage

Significant bleeding after gastric bypass has been described in 0.4% to 4% of patients. Bleeding can occur from the gastric or short gastric vessels during dissection of the greater curve. Most of the bleeding problems associated with a sleeve gastrectomy occur from the staple line after transection of the stomach. The bleeding is most likely a result of the large staples used for the thick tissue in the distal stomach. Large staples are not adequate to seal small vessels. This has led many surgeons to reinforce the staple line by over-sewing, buttressing, or both. [14]

Early bleeding typically can also occur from an anastomosis; more commonly, intraluminal bleeding occurs. Patients frequently present with tachycardia, a decreased hematocrit, and melena. Such bleeding typically resolves without surgical intervention, but may require transfusion of blood products and reversal of anticoagulation. Careful endoscopic examination and therapy is appropriate for ongoing bleeding with high transfusion requirements. Surgery is reserved for hemodynamic instability, intraluminal bleeding not amenable to endoscopic therapy (eg, staple line of the excluded stomach), or continued bleeding despite restoration of normal coagulation status. [15,16]

Venous Thromboembolism/Pulmonary Embolism

The overall incidence of a venous thromboembolism (VTE)/pulmonary embolism (PE) is approximately 0.4%. The incidence is around 0.3% for laparoscopic procedures and 1.2% for open procedures.

The most common risk factors associated with fatal PE include severe venous stasis disease, BMI >60, truncal obesity, and obesity-hypoventilation syndrome. [17]

Optimal strategies for preventing VTE/PE in the bariatric surgery setting have not been established. Most bariatric surgeons use both pneumatic compression devices in conjunction with subcutaneous unfractionated or low molecular weight heparin. The current American Society of Bariatric and Metabolic Surgeons (ASMBS) guidelines regarding VTE prophylaxis state that all bariatric patients receive mechanical prophylaxis and are ordered for early ambulation. Additionally, the surgeon may routinely use chemical prophylaxis of either low molecular weight heparin or unfractionated heparin. [18]

Preoperative risk stratification may be a useful tool for identifying high-risk patients for more aggressive prophylaxis. In patients identified preoperatively as high risk for PE, due to previous medical history of VTE, PE, or venous stasis disease, or inability to ambulate (ie, wheelchair-bound), perioperative chemoprophylaxis of low molecular weight heparin or unfractionated heparin may be prescribed for an extended period even after discharge from the hospital. [19]

Myocardial Infarction

The incidence of a postoperative MI after a bariatric operation is approximately 0.2%. [1]

Pulmonary Complications

Major postoperative pulmonary complications include pneumonia and acute respiratory failure. Atelectasis is common after all types of surgery that require general anesthesia, and is more prevalent in the morbidly obese. The overall incidence of postoperative pneumonia is around 0.4%. The overall rate of acute respiratory failure (ARF) is 1.3%. The incidence is higher with an open compared with a laparoscopic procedure, gastric bypass procedures compared with restrictive procedures and for patients with preoperative heart failure, chronic renal failure, peripheral vascular disease, chronic obstructive pulmonary disease (COPD), tobacco smoking, and diabetes. ARF is associated with a significantly higher in-hospital mortality rate compared with those who do not develop the complication.

Early ambulation and incentive spirometry after surgery are important to decrease the incidence of pulmonary complications. Preoperative identification of the presence of significant obstructive sleep apnea and initiation of continuous positive airway pressure (CPAP) therapy also reduce the risk of pulmonary complications in the postoperative period. CPAP should be used in the early postoperative period if it is clinically necessary. [20]

Surgical Site Infections

Surgical site infections (SSIs), which often are localized to the incision but can extend into deeper tissues, are the most common nosocomial infection, and are found in 2% to 5% of surgical operations in the United States. SSIs are associated with substantial morbidity, mortality, prolonged hospital stay, and increased cost of care. An overall incidence of SSIs of 1.1% has been described for bariatric surgery. Rates of wound infection are significantly greater for open procedures (10 – 15%) compared with laparoscopic (3 - 4%) procedures. Among laparoscopic techniques, rates of wound infection vary depending upon the technique used, with a higher rate of wound infections associated with the use of circular stapling devices to create the gastrojejunostomy. [21]

Signs of wound infections include unexplained fever, fluctuance, erythema, or drainage. Treatment consists of opening the affected area for drainage of infected fluid or pus, debridement of any devitalized tissue, and antibiotics if the surrounding skin suggests signs of cellulitis. The incidence of SSIs can be decreased by perioperative administration of antibiotics. [22]

In-Hospital Mortality

The intra-operative mortality is dependent upon multiple factors, including the technical difficulty of selected procedure (for example, BPD-DS technically more difficult than LAGB), patient selection (eg, body habitus), presence of comorbid illnesses (eg, COPD, congestive heart failure), skill of the surgeon (learning versus expert), institutional resources, and volume of procedures performed. While there are limited data available, the overall intra-operative mortality rates that are reported as well as the overall in-hospital mortality rates are typically <1% in most contemporary series. [23]

Pulmonary embolism (PE) remains the most common cause of mortality in the perioperative period after bariatric surgery, and accounts for approximately 30 – 50% of deaths. The mortality rate of a pulmonary embolism is dependent upon the severity of presentation and time to diagnosis/treatment, and widely varies from 1% to 95%. The majority of deaths occur within the first one to two hours after the embolism. [24]

Other common, serious causes of in-hospital mortality include cardiac events (12-17%), respiratory failure (11%), and septic complications related to an anastomotic leak (15%). [24]

30 Days Morbidity and Mortality

Early morbidity and mortality rates that occur ≤30 days after the operation are generally low and vary with surgical approach, such as fewer complications and less mortality with the laparoscopic than the open approach. Most patients have been discharged from the hospital during this one-month interval after the operation. Serious complications that occur during the in-hospital admission can also occur after discharge, such as a pulmonary embolus or myocardial infarction. The overall morbidity rate for serious complications ranges from approximately 3.4% to 12%, and varies with operative procedure (eg, RYGB, LAGB), operative approach (open versus laparoscopic), patient age, body mass index (BMI), and comorbid illnesses. The morbidity associated with LAGB appears to be less than is seen with laparoscopic Roux-en-Y gastric bypass (LRYGB). The biliopancreatic diversion with duodenal switch (BPD-DS) appears to be the riskiest procedure with the highest 30-day mortality of 1.2%, and the one associated with the most complications and highest morbidity rates. [25-26]

Marginal Ulcers

Marginal ulcers typically occur within 30 days after the RYGB operations at the gastrojejunal anastomosis and at the gastroileal junction following a BPD-DS, despite bypass or removal of most of the acid secreting cells of the stomach. The risk of a marginal ulcer following bariatric operations varies between 1.2%and 12%. The clinical presentation of marginal ulcers includes melena, hematochezia, hematemesis, or pain and obstructive symptoms as the swollen mucosa can occlude the anastomosis to the small intestine. Early ulceration most likely is related to ischemia, too large of a pouch, or undiagnosed *Helicobacter pylori* (*H. pylori*) infection. [27]

Risk factors for late presentation of a marginal ulcer include smoking, nonsteroidal antiinflammatory drugs (NSAID), or gastrogastric fistula formation. Lifetime avoidance of smoking and NSAIDS is advised. If NSAIDS are necessary, a concomitant use of a proton pump inhibitor is advised. [28]

Stenosis

Stenosis occurs when the gastrojejunal anastomosis of a RYGB or gastroileal anastomosis of a BPD-DS becomes occluded secondary to tissue edema or a narrow anastomosis. Following a LSG, stenosis can occur if the sleeve narrows, kinks, or twists. A retrospective review of 230 patients found that the risk of stenosis following a LRYGB, BPD-DS, or LSG is approximately 3.3%, 1.2%, and 3.5%, respectively. [29]

The clinical presentation is consistent with an obstruction and includes nausea, vomiting, abdominal pain, and dysphagia. Endoscopic balloon dilation of the stenotic structure is the first management option.

Stomal Obstruction

Acute stomal obstruction is an early complication that can occur in up to 14% of LAGB patients. Obstruction is usually caused by inclusion of excess perigastric fat, use of a band of insufficient diameter for the thickness of the tissue, or significant tissue edema. Patients usually present with persistent nausea, vomiting, and inability to tolerate secretions or oral intake. The diagnosis is confirmed with an upper gastrointestinal series demonstrating no passage of contrast beyond the band.

Acute stomal obstruction due to edema can initially be treated conservatively with nasogastric tube decompression until the edema subsides, although a potential for aspiration pneumonia and gastric ischemia exists. Persistent obstruction requires surgical revision or removal of the band. Meticulous removal of excess perigastric fat at the time of initial band placement may help prevent this complication. The use of larger diameter bands may also help to reduce the incidence of acute postoperative obstruction. [30]

30 Days Mortality

The overall 30-day postoperative mortality rate is generally less than 1% in most contemporary series. Mortality rates are higher for patients undergoing more complex operative procedures, or who sustain adverse intra-operative events or serious in-hospital complications (such as PE or acute respiratory failure [ARF]) as well as those with a BMI $\geq$50 kg/m^2, older age, and medical comorbidities. the mortality rate was greater for patients undergoing an open procedure compared with a laparoscopic procedure (0.79% versus 0.17%). The most common causes of death varied with the series but generally include pulmonary embolism, sepsis, complications of anastomotic leak, cardiac events, and small bowel obstruction.

Specific risk factors for mortality are male gender, older age (>65 years), excessive obesity (BMI $\geq$50 kg/m^2), comorbid illnesses, poor functional status, low-volume surgeons and hospitals (<100 procedures/year). [31,32]

Late Complications

Complications of bariatric surgery that occur after 30 days include cholelithiasis, nutritional deficiencies, and neurologic and psychiatric complications.

Cholelithiasis

Cholelithiasis develops in as many as 38% of patients within six months of surgery, and up to 41% of such patients become symptomatic. Rapid weight loss can also contribute to the development of gallstones by increasing the lithogenicity of bile. The high frequency of cholelithiasis can be reduced to as low as 2% percent with a six month course of ursodeoxycholic acid given prophylactically after weight-loss surgery. The decision to perform a cholecystectomy at the time of bariatric surgery is controversial. Some surgeons recommend performing cholecystectomy at the same time if a patient has symptomatic gallstones preoperatively. The surgical opinion about asymptomatic gallstones is more divided, and studies have failed to demonstrate a benefit for simultaneous cholecystectomy for incidental gallstones.

Patients can also develop choledocholithiasis, which can be difficult to treat in the postoperative course of RYGB. Diagnosis of choledocholithiasis can be confirmed by ultrasound or magnetic resonance cholangiopancreatography (MRCP); however, endoscopic intervention and management can be difficult because of the relative inaccessibility to the duodenum due to the altered anatomy of the Roux-en-Y configuration. As a result, successful endoscopic retrograde cholangiopancreatography (ERCP) with cannulation of the papilla is very difficult to perform. Thus, treatment of choledocholithiasis may require surgery or transhepatic percutaneous access. [33, 34]

Ventral Incisional Hernia

Ventral incisional hernias occur with a frequency of 0 - 1.8% in laparoscopic series and as high as 24% in open series, underscoring a clear advantage of the laparoscopic approach in this regard. Incisional hernias present with an enlarging bulge, pain, or obstructive symptoms. Severe obesity is associated with increased intra-abdominal pressure and thus, a high risk of hernia development after a laparotomy. Many surgeons postpone a formal repair until significant weight loss occurs (>1 year). Indications for early surgical repair include significant pain, bowel obstruction, and rapid enlargement of the hernia. [35]

Complications of Specific Bariatric Procedures

Roux-En-Y Gastric Bypass

Gastric Remnant Distension

Gastric remnant distension is a rare but potentially lethal complication following gastric bypass. The gastric remnant is a blind pouch and may become distended if paralytic ileus or distal mechanical obstruction occurs postoperatively. Iatrogenic injury to vagal fibers along the lesser curvature may also contribute, possibly by leading to impaired emptying of the bypassed stomach. Progressive distension can ultimately lead to rupture, spillage of massive gastric contents, and subsequent severe peritonitis. The combination of the large size of inoculum (liters) and the injurious contents (acid, bile, pancreatic enzymes, and bacteria) makes this complication much more serious than leakage occurring at the gastrojejunostomy.

Clinical features include pain, hiccups, left upper quadrant tympany, shoulder pain, abdominal distension, tachycardia, or shortness of breath. Radiographic assessment may demonstrate a large gastric air bubble.

Treatment consists of emergent operative decompression with a gastrostomy tube or percutaneous gastrostomy. Immediate operative exploration and decompression are required if percutaneous drainage is not feasible, or if perforation is suspected. Although gastrostomy is not performed routinely by most surgeons at the initial gastric bypass operation, drainage of the gastric remnant can prevent this rare but sometimes fatal complication. Routine gastrostomy should be considered in the elderly, super-obese patients, patients with diabetic gastropathy and as part of revisional surgeries where gastric emptying may be delayed. [36]

Dumping Syndrome

Dumping syndrome can occur in up to 50% of postgastric bypass patients when high levels of simple carbohydrates are ingested. Dumping may contribute to weight loss in part by causing the patient to modify the eating habits.

There are two types of dumping syndrome: early and late. [37]

- Early dumping syndrome — Early dumping syndrome has a rapid onset, usually within 15 minutes. It is the result of rapid emptying of food into the small bowel. Due to the hyperosmolality of the food, rapid fluid shifts from the plasma into the bowel occur, resulting in hypotension and a sympathetic nervous system response. Patients often present with colicky abdominal pain, diarrhea, nausea, and tachycardia. Patients should avoid foods that are high in simple sugar content and replace them with a diet consisting of high fiber, complex carbohydrate, and protein rich foods. Behavioral modification, such as small, frequent meals, and separating solids from liquid intake by 30 minutes, are also advocated. Usually, early dumping is self-limiting and resolves within 7 to 12 weeks.
- Late dumping syndrome — Late dumping syndrome is a result of the hyperglycemia and the subsequent insulin response leading to hypoglycemia that occurs 2 to 3 hours after a meal. Patients present with dizziness, fatigue, diaphoresis and weakness. The treatment is similar to early dumping syndrome.

Metabolic and Nutritional Derangements

Metabolic and nutritional derangements are common in severely obese patients and can be exacerbated following after bariatric surgery, making postoperative life-long compliance with appropriate dietary choices and vitamin supplementation imperative. Decreased oral intake as well as altered absorption of food from the stomach and small bowel reduces absorption of various micronutrients, particularly iron, calcium, vitamin B12, thiamine and folate. Hyperoxaluria and nephrolithiasis have been reported following Roux-en-Y gastric bypass surgery.

Change in Bowel Habits

Loss stool and diarrhea are more common after BPD and RYGB. Constipation is more common after gastric banding. Steatorrhea and more frequent stools can occur with excessive fat intake. In addition, these symptoms can be due to subclinical lactose intolerance, which is only recognized when dairy products are used in an effort to achieve adequate protein intake after bariatric surgery. [38]

Failure to Lose Weight and Weight Regain

Failure to lose weight following Roux-en-Y gastric bypass is rare, and is often due to maladaptive eating patterns during the early postoperative period. On the other hand, significant late weight regain occurs in up to 20% of patients, especially those with super-obesity (BMI >50 kg/m2) at the time of the initial operation. It is often due to progressive noncompliant eating and other behavioral habits, development of a functional gastrogastric fistula, gradual enlargement of the gastric pouch, or dilatation of the gastrojejunal anastomosis. [39]

Gastric Banding

Band Erosion

Band erosion through the wall of the stomach has been reported in up to 7% of GB patients, and it is thought to occur as a result of either gastric wall ischemia from an excessively tight band, mechanical trauma related to the band buckle or thermal trauma from electrosurgical energy sources used during band placement. Band erosion is a late complication and occurs at a mean of 22 months after surgery.

Clinical signs of band erosion include infection, failure of weight loss, or nausea and vomiting. Epigastric pain and hematemesis can also signal erosion of the lap band into the left gastric artery. This can happen when the lap band erodes into the posterior part of the stomach near the cardioesophageal junction. This complication can be avoided by careful placement during the initial surgery, making sure not to include the ascending branch of the left gastric artery during band placement.

Band erosion can be diagnosed by endoscopy and treatment involves removal of the band, which can be done laparoscopically. It is generally recommended that revision to another bariatric procedure be delayed for at least 2 to 3 months after an episode of band erosion, as the complication rate with immediate revision is increased. [40]

Band Slippage and Gastric Prolapse

Band slippage involves prolapse of part of the stomach through the band, with varying degrees of gastric obstruction. Slippage rates can be as high as 24%.

- Anterior prolapse involves migration of the band cephalad which creates an acute angle with the stomach pouch and esophagus, resulting in obstruction.
- Posterior gastric prolapse occurs when the stomach migrates cephalad, displacing the band caudally and creating a new pouch

Gastric prolapse is characterized by food intolerance, epigastric pain, and acid reflux. Diagnosis is confirmed with an upper gastrointestinal series demonstrating either malposition of the band or dilatation and prolapse of the gastric pouch.

Surgery is required urgently or emergently, depending on the presentation. Repair of the prolapse can sometimes be accomplished by repositioning the band, but often the band needs to be replaced or removed altogether, especially if significant inflammation is found. [41]

Port Malfunction

Port malfunction results if the tubing disconnects, subcutaneous port flips, or leakage within the system occurs. Such problems lead to inability to titrate the instilled volume of saline in the system. Reported incidence of port and tubing malfunction ranges from 0.4% to 7%. These problems usually become evident as an inability to access port and maintain band volume, or the development of weight gain. These complications require surgical repair or exchange of the hardware to attain band adjustability. Port dislocation can be reduced by attaching the port to a broad surface mesh first before anchoring to the rectus fascia. [42]

Esophagitis

Esophagitis and reflux are infrequent complications following Lap-Band. Deflation of the band and acid-suppression therapy are the mainstays of treatment. However, if intractable to medical therapy, band removal or conversion to other procedure such as RYGB may be necessary. [43]

Esophageal Dilatation

Esophageal dilatation proximal to the band device has been observed in as many as 10% of patients. This so-called "pseudoachalasia syndrome" may develop when the band is excessively inflated or in the setting of excessive amounts of food intake. Pouch dilatation has also been associated with a history of binge eating behavior. Patients often present with food and saliva intolerance, reflux and epigastric discomfort. The diagnosis can be confirmed with an upper gastrointestinal series.

The initial treatment should be removal of all the fluid from the band and behavioral diet modifications. This is usually successful in reversing esophageal dilatation. However, persistent dilatation may require replacement of the band in a new location on the stomach or conversion to a different procedure.

Deflation of the band alone is usually successful in reversing esophageal dilatation. However, persistent dilatation may require replacement of the band to a new location on the stomach or conversion to a different procedure. [44]

Hiatus Hernia

Hiatus hernia is often a pre-existing but unrecognized condition in patients undergoing bariatric surgery**.** This can lead to ongoing intractable reflux necessitating reoperation or band removal. Thus, a simple crural repair can be performed at the initial operation to avoid these complications. [45]

Sleeve Gastrectomy

Bleeding

Bleeding can occur from the gastric or short gastric vessels during dissection of the greater curve. Most of the bleeding problems associated with SG occur from the staple line after transection of the stomach. The bleeding is most likely a result of the large staples used for the thick tissue in the distal stomach. Large staples are not adequate to seal small vessels. This has led many surgeons to reinforce the staple line by over-sewing, buttressing or both. [46]

Stenosis

Narrowing or stenosis can create gastric outlet obstruction. The presentation varies depending on the severity of the obstruction and can include dysphagia, vomiting, dehydration and the inability to tolerate an oral diet.

The gastroesophageal junction and the incisura angularis are the two most common areas where stenosis occurs, and this can be diagnosed by an upper gastrointestinal series.

The most common reasons for the development of narrowing or stenosis are over-sewing the staple line and using a bougie that is too small. The preferable bougie size is currently debated in the literature and can range from 30 to 60 French. In most cases, surgeons use a 36 to 40 French bougie for the sleeve construction and the larger sizes of bougies are reserved for when SG is being performed as part of a staged procedure.

Management of stenosis primarily consists of endoscopic dilation. If the area of stenosis is too long, surgical intervention may be necessary with conversion to a RYGB, gastric stricturoplasty or resection with gastrogastrostomy. [47]

Gastric Leaks

Gastric leaks after SG are one of the most serious complications and can occur in up to 5.3% of patients.

Most leaks are due to local factors at the site of the staple line, such as inadequate blood supply and oxygenation, which impede the healing process. Leaks can also be due to gastric-wall heat ischemia, a consequence of the heat generated by the cautery used during dissection of the greater curve. Although the blood supply to the stomach is robust, the gastroesophageal junction tends to be an area of decreased vascularity and thus more prone to leaks. Additionally, the stomach tends to be thinner at the angle of His and some authors suggest that the large staple height used by many surgeons may not adequately seal this area of the stomach.

Some surgeons recommend leaving a small portion of stomach distal to the angle of His and then imbricating with a running suture. However, clinical studies have not provided evidence that reinforcing the suture line decreases the rate of leak after sleeve gastrectomy. Sleeve gastrectomy produces high intragastric pressure, which can affect the healing process and lengthen the amount of time for a leak to close. [48,49]

Reoperation with primary repair during the early postoperative course is the best option for a leak following SG. Clinically stable patients may be able to undergo percutaneous drainage, antibiotic therapy, and parenteral nutrition until the leak is healed. Endoscopic therapy with the use of stents has also been employed for management of leaks, but migration of the stents has been a problem. Early diagnosis, adequate drainage and gastric decompression are the mainstay of treatment for leaks. [50]

Reflux

Gastroesophageal reflux after SG presents with classic symptoms such as burning pain, heartburn, and regurgitation. It can occur as an early and late complication. The first-line treatment is antireflux medical therapy. GERD unresponsive to antireflux medical therapy with no clear anatomic abnormalities, such as stoma stenosis or a hiatal hernia, can be effectively treated by conversion to RYGB. [51]

Pure Malabsorptive Procedures (Biliopancreatic Diversion and Duodenal Switch)

Electrolyte Imbalances

Over half of the patients who underwent ,malabsorptive procedures developed diarrhea and electrolyte imbalances, and these problems could persist more than five years after surgery. Arthritis, protein malnutrition, vitamin deficiencies, cirrhosis, nephrolithiasis with oxalate stones and renal failure have also been associated. [52]

Renal Failure

Increased absorption of calcium oxalate leads to deposition in the renal parenchyma. This can lead to a postobstruction nephropathy and renal failure, which has been described in up to 20% of patients. Conversion to a gastric bypass or reversal should be considered in patients with metabolic complications. [53]

Cirrhosis

Hepatic abnormalities that may lead to cirrhosis can occur in up to 40% of patients and may persist or progress despite reversal in more than one-third of patients. Some patients have progressed to decompensated cirrhosis requiring transplantation. Progressive liver injury appears histologically as increasing steatosis, lobular lymphocytic inflammation, pericellular fibrosis, Mallory bodies, and deranged architecture, all features resembling those seen in alcoholic liver disease. [54]

Improvement of Comorbidities

Weight Loss

Excess Body Weight

Excess body weight is defined as the amount of weight that is in excess of the ideal body weight. Ideal body weight is conventionally determined by the body mass index (BMI) <25 kg/m^2.

Based upon prospective studies and a randomized trial, the rate of weight loss varies with the specific bariatric procedures, as illustrated:

- For patients undergoing a Roux-en-Y Gastric Bypass (RYGB) or a sleeve gastrectomy (SG), weight loss occurs rapidly over the first few months, then continues over the next year to year and a half until weight loss reaches a plateau. During the first six months after RYGB, the average weight loss is 4.5 to 7 kg per month. Thus, average weight loss at the six-month follow up visit is 27 to 36 kg. Thereafter, the rate of weight loss tends to slow down to 2 to 3 kg per month, and total weight loss reaches a peak at 12 months postoperatively, averaging 45 to 54 kg.
- For patients who undergo an adjustable gastric band (AGB) procedure, weight loss is slower, with an anticipated one pound per week weight loss until stabilization is reached at approximately two years. Although most patients do well initially, some

ultimately fail to sustain their improvement. Some AGB patients may not ever achieve significant weight loss. This highlights the importance of establishing a fundamental life-style change during the first one to two years after surgery in order to achieve long-term success in maintaining weight loss. [55-57]

Medical Comorbidities

Diabetes Mellitus

Bariatric surgical procedures are effective interventions for treating type 2 diabetes. Improvement in metabolic control is often evident within days to weeks following bariatric procedures, most likely reflecting an alteration in metabolism that is independent of weight loss. [58]

Three randomized trials illustrate the efficacy of weight loss surgery versus medical therapy alone:

- Obese patients with uncontrolled type II diabetes undergoing a RYGB or a SG plus medical therapy were significantly more likely to achieve the main outcome of a glycated hemoglobin level of 6.0 percent or less at 12 months compared with patients managed by intensive medical therapy alone (42% versus 37% versus 12%, respectively). [59]
- A randomized trial of 60 patients also found that obese diabetic patients undergoing a bariatric operation had better control than medical management alone. Obese patients (BMI ≥35) with a history of diabetes for five or more years and a glycated hemoglobin level ≥7.0 percent undergoing a RYGB or biliopancreatic diversion (BPD) were significantly more likely to achieve the study endpoint of remission of diabetes at two years compared with patients managed by medical therapy alone (75% versus 95% versus 0%, respectively). [60]
- A randomized trial that included 120 patients demonstrated that a RYGB procedure was superior to intensive medical management alone in achieving the main outcome measure of a glycated hemoglobin level of less than 7%. (75% versus 32%). [61]

Results following RYGB operation are promising and several trials are in progress to evaluate the procedure for patients with BMI <35 and poorly controlled type 2 diabetes. [62,63] Efficacious control of type 2 diabetes has also been demonstrated following a SG or an AGB.

In 2011, the American College of Surgeons Bariatric Surgery Center Network (ACS-BSCN) found that the remission or improvement was for patients undergoing RYGB, SG, and AGB. In a prospective, longitudinal study that included bariatric-specific data from more than 100 participating institutions and 28,616 obese diabetic patients, remission or improvement in diabetes at 12 months was achieved in 83 percent of patients undergoing a RYGB, 55 percent undergoing SG, and 44 percent undergoing an AGB. [64] This result has been corroborated by other studies demonstrating one-year remission or improvement of diabetes in 40% to 75% of patients who underwent a SG or an AGB. [27,28,65,66]. SG is an alternative procedure to RYGB for patients with BMI <50, the extremes of ages, and smokers.

In addition to glycemic control, improvement in distal peripheral neuropathy was identified following RYGB. An improvement or normalization of the Neuropathy Symptom Score (NSS) and the Neuropathy Deficit Score (NDS) in all patients has been found. [67]

Hypertension

The association between obesity and the development of hypertension is well established. Weight loss, whether by an intensive lifestyle-medical modification program or a bariatric operation, improves obesity-linked hypertension or contributes to remission. Patients undergoing a bariatric surgery plus intensive lifestyle medical management were able to achieve a similar reduction in systolic blood pressure at 12 months compared with patients managed with lifestyle medical modification alone. [68] While intensive lifestyle modification resulting in weight loss appears beneficial for resolution of hypertension, this is unfortunately not feasible for all patients, due to reasons such as lack of motivation or inability to exercise.

Data are unclear as to whether or not RYGB offers the highest resolution or reduction of hypertension of bariatric operations, as illustrated by several studies. [64,69]

Dyslipidemia

Obesity-linked dyslipidemia is a well-established risk factor for cardiovascular disease. [70]. The most commonly encountered dyslipidemias in obese individuals include hypertriglyceridemia, decreased HDL-cholesterol values, and increased LDL-cholesterol particles. [71] Multiple studies have demonstrated improved lipid profiles following bariatric procedures. The most extensively studied procedure is the RYGB. Mean total cholesterol levels decreased by 16%, triglyceride levels decreased by 63%, LDL- cholesterol levels decreased by 31%, total cholesterol/HDL-cholesterol risk ratio decreased by 60%, and HDL-cholesterol levels increased by 39%. In addition, over 80% of patients requiring lipid-lowering medications preoperatively no longer required medical therapy. [72] Malabsorptive procedures obtain at least similar results of improvement of dyslipidemia. A recent study of our group has demonstrated that after SG, HDL-cholesterol values increase and Triglycerides levels decreased significantly. However, total and LDL-cholesterol remained unaltered of present nonsignificant improvements. Notwithstanding, mainly based on the HDL-cholesterol increase, the cardiovascular risk index present a significant improvement after surgery. [73]

Obstructive Sleep Apnea

An increased prevalence of obstructive sleep apnea in the obese population is well established. [74] Weight loss decreases apnea hypopnea index (AHI, the number of apneas and hypopneas per hour of sleep). In addition, weight loss achieved from bariatric operations also reduces AHI and appears to be similar to the efficacy of behavioral modification weight loss. However, a meta-analysis of 69 studies performed in 2013 identified a high rate of resolution or improvement in OSA following bariatric procedures. [75]

Gastroesophageal Reflux Disease

Obesity is a well-established risk factor for the development of gastroesophageal reflux disease (GERD). The impact of bariatric surgery on development, resolution, or exacerbation of GERD is an evolving topic of debate. Improvement of GERD may be dependent upon the type of bariatric procedure performed. RYGB may improve or ameliorate GERD symptoms. In addition, there is a significant improvement in esophagitis, presence of extraesophageal syndromes, use of proton pump inhibitors, and decreased total acid exposure. [76]

There are conflicting and inconclusive data on the association between AGB and prevalence of postoperative GERD. A systematic review that included 20 studies and 3307 obese patients undergoing AGB found a decrease in prevalence of postoperative GERD compared with the prevalence of preoperative one (7.7% versus 32.9%. In addition, the rate of use of anti-reflux medications decreased in the AGB postoperative period, the prevalence of pathologic reflux also decreased in the postoperative period, and the lower esophageal pressures improved after AGB. However, reflux symptoms developed in the postoperative period in 15% of patients who were asymptomatic preoperatively, and the rate of esophageal dysmotility increased following AGB. Based upon this review, it appears that AGB may have anti-reflux properties for some obese patients, but the procedure may also be associated with the development or worsening of reflux symptoms. [77]

While also highly debated, SG may be the least efficacious procedure to reduce postoperative GERD. In a systematic review of 11 prospective and retrospective studies that included 1058 patients, seven studies identified a decrease in GERD prevalence and four studies found an increase in GERD. [78] This lack of consensus regarding the association between SG and GERD was again reiterated during the 2011 International Sleeve Gastrectomy Expert Panel Consensus Statement where no consensus was reached regarding performance of sleeve gastrectomy in patients with gastric reflux. [79] Based on these data, we consider that preoperative GERD is a relative contraindication for undergoing a SG and in such cases we prefer performing a RYGB. [73]

Polycystic Ovary Syndrome

Polycystic ovarian syndrome (PCOS) is found in 30% to 70% of obese women of reproductive age and is associated with a high risk of infertility. [80] Weight reduction through diet and exercise and lifestyle modification can improve the hyperandrogenemic symptoms and insulin resistance associated with PCOS. Bariatric surgery is an alternative strategy for weight loss in women with PCOS. Obese women who effectively achieved weight loss following a RYGB had restored menstrual cycles at approximately three to four months following the operation, marked lessening of hirsutism and hyperandrogenemia at eight months, and an increased ability to conceive within two years of surgery.Similar studies have not been published for adjustable gastric band or sleeve gastrectomy. [81, 82]

Oncologic

The association between obesity and certain cancers, such as breast, endometrial, colon, renal, and pancreatic cancers has been well established. Obesity also increases the likelihood of worse oncologic outcomes. The impact of bariatric surgery on oncologic outcome is difficult to assess in a short-term time frame, as longer time intervals are necessary to establish true risk reduction. [83-85]

Nonalcoholic Fatty Liver Disease (NAFLD)

Nonalcoholic fatty liver disease (NAFLD) is one of the most common causes of chronic liver disease worldwide, and morbid obesity is strongly associated with its development. [86]

NAFLD is subdivided into nonalcoholic fatty liver (NAFL), hepatic steatosis without inflammation, and nonalcoholic steatohepatitis (NASH), which is associated with inflammation and can be indistinguishable histologically from alcoholic steatohepatitis.

The general approach to the overweight or obese patient with NAFLD or NASH is lifestyle modification and weight loss. [87] Histologic improvement has also been observed in some patients with NAFLD or NASH after bariatric surgery. At this time, it is not advised to perform a bariatric operation specifically for the purpose of improving NAFLD or NASH, nor is the optimal bariatric procedure yet identified. Given the potential for worsening fibrosis in some patients following bariatric surgery, patients should continue to have liver function tests monitored closely. [88]

Psychosocial Effect and Impact on Quality of Life

Psychological Impact

Effective outcomes following bariatric surgery include psychosocial improvements. [89] There is a general tendency for patients with psychopathologic disorders to improve or normalize after bariatric surgery. [89-93] This may occur because patients take an active role in changing their lives, even while they are still overweight. [94-95]

- A prospective study that included 200 patients undergoing gastric bypass surgery found postoperative improvement at 20, 40, and 92 weeks in health-related (Short-Form 36) and weight-related (Impact of Weight on Quality of Life) quality of life surveys compared with the preoperative responses. [96]
- The Body Shape Questionnaire (BSQ) measures preoccupation with one's body shape and the Shape and Weight Concern subscales of the Eating Disorder Examination-Questionnaire (EDE-Q) assesses dissatisfaction, preoccupation, discomfort, and overvaluation of body shape. For 109 patients undergoing RYGB, responses to BSQ and EDE-Q surveys at 6 months and 12 months after RYGB were improved compared with preoperative responses. [97] In addition, over 80% of female patients had body image scores comparable with published normal values.

There are, at present, no data from prospective studies that assess the psychosocial impact of a sleeve gastrectomy (SG). Based upon the studies that show improvement with weight loss associated with RYGB and AGB, it is reasonable to surmise that patients undergoing a SG would also experience a similar benefit.

However, not all patients experience psychosocial improvement following bariatric surgery. Lack of improved psychosocial function may accompany lack of postoperative weight loss, some may initially improve but later experience declines of function even with maintenance of weight, and others lag behind functioning of normal patients. [89,92,94]

Impact on Quality of Life

Altogether, the improvement of most comorbidities associated with morbid obesity, and the increasing self-esteem based on esthetic reasons, leads to a significant improvement of the quality of life. The patients feel healthier and this has a positive psychological impact. There are many scales available to evaluate quality of life, but all of them coincide in that bariatric surgery achieves a significant improvement in the quality of life of morbidly obese patients. [92-94]

References

[1] Encinosa WE, Bernard DM, Du D, Steiner CA. Recent improvements in bariatric surgery outcomes. *Med Care* 2009; 47:531-5.

[2] Longitudinal Assessment of Bariatric Surgery (LABS) Consortium, Flum DR, Belle SH, et al. Perioperative safety in the longitudinal assessment of bariatric surgery. *N Engl J Med* 2009; 361:445-54.

[3] Lancaster RT, Hutter MM. Bands and bypasses: 30-day morbidity and mortality of bariatric surgical procedures as assessed by prospective, multi-center, risk-adjusted ACS-NSQIP data. *Surg Endosc 2008*; 22:2554-63.

[4] Ahmad G, Duffy JM, Phillips K, Watson A. Laparoscopic entry techniques. *Cochrane Database Syst Rev* 2008; :CD006583.

[5] Peters TG, Steinmetz SR, Cowan GS Jr. Splenic injury and repair during bariatric surgical procedures. *South Med J* 1990; 83:166-9.

[6] Huerta S, Li Z, Livingston EH. Outcome of portal injuries following bariatric operations. *Obes Surg* 2006; 16:105-9.

[7] Al-Khyatt W, Thomas JD, Humes DJ, Lobo DN. Intestinal ischemia following laparoscopic surgery: a case series. *J Med Case Rep* 2013; 7:25.

[8] Mitchell MT, Gasparaitis AE, Alverdy JC. Imaging findings in Roux-en-O and other misconstructions: rare but serious complications of Roux-en-Y gastric bypass surgery. AJR *Am J Roentgenol* 2008; 190:367-73.

[9] Stroh C, Köckerling F, Weiner R, et al. Are there gender-specific aspects of sleeve gastrectomy-data analysis from the quality assurance study of surgical treatment of obesity in Germany. *Obes Surg* 2012; 22:1214-9.

[10] Gentileschi P, Camperchioli I, D'Ugo S, et al. Staple-line reinforcement during laparoscopic sleeve gastrectomy using three different techniques: a randomized trial. *Surg Endosc* 2012; 26:2623-9.

[11] Lim RB, Blackburn GL, Jones DB. Benchmarking best practices in weight loss surgery. *Curr Probl Surg* 2010; 47:79-174.

[12] Madan AK, Stoecklein HH, Ternovits CA, et al. Predictive value of upper gastrointestinal studies versus clinical signs for gastrointestinal leaks after laparoscopic gastric bypass. *Surg Endosc* 2007; 21:194-6.

[13] Gonzalez R, Sarr MG, Smith CD, et al. Diagnosis and contemporary management of anastomotic leaks after gastric bypass for obesity. *J Am Coll Surg* 2007; 204:47-55.

[14] Wittgrove AC, Clark GW. Laparoscopic gastric bypass, Roux-en-Y- 500 patients: technique and results, with 3-60 month follow-up. *Obes Surg* 2000; 10:233-9.

[15] Frezza EE, Reddy S, Gee LL, Wachtel MS. Complications after sleeve gastrectomy for morbid obesity. *Obes Surg* 2009; 19:684-7.

[16] Lalor PF, Tucker ON, Szomstein S, Rosenthal RJ. Complications after laparoscopic sleeve gastrectomy. *Surg Obes Relat Dis* 2008; 4:33-8.

[17] Winegar DA, Sherif B, Pate V, DeMaria EJ. Venous thromboembolism after bariatric surgery performed by Bariatric Surgery Center of Excellence Participants: analysis of the Bariatric Outcomes Longitudinal Database. *Surg Obes Relat Dis* 2011; 7:181-8.

[18] American Society for Metabolic and Bariatric Surgery Clinical Issues Committee. ASMBS updated position statement on prophylactic measures to reduce the risk of venous thromboembolism in bariatric surgery patients. *Surg Obes Relat Dis* 2013; 9:493-7.

[19] Caruana JA, Anain PM, Pham DT. The pulmonary embolism risk score system reduces the incidence and mortality of pulmonary embolism after gastric bypass. *Surgery* 2009; 146:678-83.

[20] Masoomi H, Reavis KM, Smith BR, et al. Risk factors for acute respiratory failure in bariatric surgery: data from the Nationwide Inpatient Sample, 2006-2008. *Surg Obes Relat Dis* 2013; 9:277-81.

[21] Nelson DW, Blair KS, Martin MJ. Analysis of obesity-related outcomes and bariatric failure rates with the duodenal switch vs gastric bypass for morbid obesity. *Arch Surg* 2012; 147:847-54.

[22] Bohdjalian A, Langer FB, Kranner A, et al. Circular- vs. linear-stapled gastrojejunostomy in laparoscopic Roux-en-Y gastric bypass. *Obes Surg* 2010; 20:440-6.

[23] Buchwald H, Avidor Y, Braunwald E, et al. Bariatric surgery: a systematic review and meta-analysis. *JAMA* 2004; 292:1724-37.

[24] Stephens DJ, Saunders JK, Belsley S, et al. Short-term outcomes for super-super obese (BMI > or =60 kg/m2) patients undergoing weight loss surgery at a high-volume bariatric surgery center: laparoscopic adjustable gastric banding, laparoscopic gastric bypass, and open tubular gastric bypass. *Surg Obes Relat Dis* 2008; 4:408-15.

[25] Blackstone RP, Cortés MC. Metabolic acuity score: effect on major complications after bariatric surgery. *Surg Obes Relat Dis* 2010;6:267-73.

[26] Prachand VN, Davee RT, Alverdy JC. Duodenal switch provides superior weight loss in the super-obese (BMI > or =50 kg/m2) compared with gastric bypass. *Ann Surg.* 2006;244:611-9.

[27] Csendes A, Burgos AM, Altuve J, Bonacic S. Incidence of marginal ulcer 1 month and 1 to 2 years after gastric bypass: a prospective consecutive endoscopic evaluation of 442 patients with morbid obesity. *Obes Surg* 2009; 19:135-8.

[28] Azagury DE, Abu Dayyeh BK, Greenwalt IT, Thompson CC. Marginal ulceration after Roux-en-Y gastric bypass surgery: characteristics, risk factors, treatment, and outcomes. *Endoscopy* 2011; 43:950-4.

[29] Parikh A, Alley JB, Peterson RM, et al. Management options for symptomatic stenosis after laparoscopic vertical sleeve gastrectomy in the morbidly obese. *Surg Endosc* 2012; 26:738-46.

[30] Gravante G, Araco A, Araco F, et al. Laparoscopic adjustable gastric bandings: a prospective randomized study of 400 operations performed with 2 different devices. *Arch Surg* 2007; 142:958-61.

[31] Ballantyne GH, Belsley S, Stephens D, et al. Bariatric surgery: low mortality at a high-volume center. *Obes Surg* 2008; 18:660-7.

[32] Nguyen NT, Masoomi H, Laugenour K, et al. Predictive factors of mortality in bariatric surgery: data from the Nationwide Inpatient Sample. *Surgery* 2011; 150:347-51.
[33] Villegas L, Schneider B, Provost D, et al. Is routine cholecystectomy required during laparoscopic gastric bypass? *Obes Surg* 2004; 14:206-11.
[34] Hamad GG, Ikramuddin S, Gourash WF, Schauer PR. Elective cholecystectomy during laparoscopic Roux-en-Y gastric bypass: is it worth the wait? *Obes Surg* 2003; 13:76-81.
[35] Lee S, Carmody B, Wolfe L, et al. Effect of location and speed of diagnosis on anastomotic leak outcomes in 3828 gastric bypass cases. *J Gastrointest Surg* 2007; 11:708-13.
[36] Nguyen NT, Ho HS, Palmer LS, Wolfe BM. A comparison study of laparoscopic versus open gastric bypass for morbid obesity. *J Am Coll Surg* 2000; 191:149-55.
[37] Ukleja A. Dumping syndrome: pathophysiology and treatment. *Nutr Clin Pract* 2005; 20:517-25.
[38] Potoczna N, Harfmann S, Steffen R, et al. Bowel habits after bariatric surgery. *Obes Surg* 2008; 18:1287-96.
[39] Kalarchian MA, Marcus MD, Wilson GT, et al. Binge eating among gastric bypass patients at long-term follow-up. *Obes Surg* 2002; 12:270-5.
[40] Brown WA, Egberts KJ, Franke-Richard D, et al. Erosions after laparoscopic adjustable gastric banding: diagnosis and management. *Ann Surg* 2013; 257:1047-52.
[41] Abuzeid AW, Banerjea A, Timmis B, Hashemi M. Gastric slippage as an emergency: diagnosis and management. *Obes Surg* 2007; 17:559-61.
[42] Fabry H, Van Hee R, Hendrickx L, Totté E. A technique for prevention of port complications after laparoscopic adjustable silicone gastric banding. *Obes Surg* 2002; 12:285-8.
[43] Rubenstein RB. Laparoscopic adjustable gastric banding at a U.S. center with up to 3-year follow-up. *Obes Surg* 2002; 12:380-4.
[44] Poole N, Al Atar A, Bidlake L, et al. Pouch dilatation following laparoscopic adjustable gastric banding: psychobehavioral factors (can psychiatrists predict pouch dilatation?). *Obes Surg* 2004; 14:798-801.
[45] Gulkarov I, Wetterau M, Ren CJ, Fielding GA. Hiatal hernia repair at the initial laparoscopic adjustable gastric band operation reduces the need for reoperation. *Surg Endosc* 2008; 22:1035-41.
[46] Frezza EE, Reddy S, Gee LL, Wachtel MS. Complications after sleeve gastrectomy for morbid obesity. *Obes Surg* 2009; 19:684-7.
[47] Dapri G, Cadière GB, Himpens J. Laparoscopic seromyotomy for long stenosis after sleeve gastrectomy with or without duodenal switch. *Obes Surg* 2009; 19:495-9.
[48] Arias E, Martínez PR, Ka Ming Li V, et al. Mid-term follow-up after sleeve gastrectomy as a final approach for morbid obesity. *Obes Surg* 2009; 19:544-8.
[49] Burgos AM, Braghetto I, Csendes A, et al. Gastric leak after laparoscopic-sleeve gastrectomy for obesity. *Obes Surg* 2009; 19:1672-7.
[50] Oshiro T, Kasama K, Umezawa A, et al. Successful management of refractory staple line leakage at the esophagogastric junction after a sleeve gastrectomy using the HANAROSTENT. *Obes Surg* 2010; 20:530-4.
[51] Langer FB, Bohdjalian A, Shakeri-Leidenmühler S, et al. Conversion from sleeve gastrectomy to Roux-en-Y gastric bypass--indications and outcome. *Obes Surg* 2010; 20:835-40.

[52] Markowitz JS, Seu P, Goss JA, et al. Liver transplantation for decompensated cirrhosis after jejunoileal bypass: a strategy for management. *Transplantation* 1998; 65:570-2.

[53] Requarth JA, Burchard KW, Colacchio TA, et al. Long-term morbidity following jejunoileal bypass. The continuing potential need for surgical reversal. *Arch Surg* 1995; 130:318-25.

[54] Dean P, Joshi S, Kaminski DL. Long-term outcome of reversal of small intestinal bypass operations. *Am J Surg* 1990; 159:118-23.

[55] BMI classification. World Health Organization. apps.who.int/bmi/index.jsp?intro Page=intro_3.html (Accessed on August 29, 2013).

[56] Cunneen SA. Review of meta-analytic comparisons of bariatric surgery with a focus on laparoscopic adjustable gastric banding. *Surg Obes Relat Dis.* 2008;4:S47-55.

[57] Ballantyne GH. Measuring outcomes following bariatric surgery: weight loss parameters, improvement in co-morbid conditions, change in quality of life and patient satisfaction. *Obes Surg* 2003; 13:954-64.

[58] Rubino F. Is type 2 diabetes an operable intestinal disease? A provocative yet reasonable hypothesis. *Diabetes Care* 2008; 31 Suppl 2:S290-6.

[59] Schauer PR, Kashyap SR, Wolski K, et al. Bariatric surgery versus intensive medical therapy in obese patients with diabetes. *N Engl J Med* 2012; 366:1567-76.

[60] Mingrone G, Panunzi S, De Gaetano A, et al. Bariatric surgery versus conventional medical therapy for type 2 diabetes. *N Engl J Med* 2012; 366:1577-85.

[61] Ikramuddin S, Korner J, Lee WJ, et al. Roux-en-Y gastric bypass vs intensive medical management for the control of type 2 diabetes, hypertension, and hyperlipidemia: the Diabetes Surgery Study randomized clinical trial. *JAMA* 2013; 309:2240.-9

[62] Rubino F, Kaplan LM, Schauer PR, et al. The Diabetes Surgery Summit consensus conference: recommendations for the evaluation and use of gastrointestinal surgery to treat type 2 diabetes mellitus. *Ann Surg* 2010; 251:399-405.

[63] Kenngott HG, Clemens G, Gondan M, et al. DiaSurg 2 trial - surgical vs. medical treatment of insulin-dependent type 2 diabetes mellitus in patients with a body mass index between 26 and 35 kg/m2: study protocol of a randomized controlled multicenter trial - DRKS00004550. *Trials* 2013; 14:183.

[64] Hutter MM, Schirmer BD, Jones DB, et al. First report from the American College of Surgeons Bariatric Surgery Center Network: laparoscopic sleeve gastrectomy has morbidity and effectiveness positioned between the band and the bypass. *Ann Surg* 2011; 254:410-20.

[65] Dixon JB, O'Brien PE, Playfair J, et al. Adjustable gastric banding and conventional therapy for type 2 diabetes: a randomized controlled trial. *JAMA* 2008; 299:316-23.

[66] Ahn SM, Pomp A, Rubino F. Metabolic surgery for type 2 diabetes. *Ann N Y Acad Sci* 2010; 1212:E37-45.

[67] Müller-Stich BP, Fischer L, Kenngott HG, et al. Gastric bypass leads to improvement of diabetic neuropathy independent of glucose normalization--results of a prospective cohort study (DiaSurg 1 study). *Ann Surg* 2013; 258:760-5.

[68] Ikramuddin S, Korner J, Lee WJ, et al. Roux-en-Y gastric bypass vs intensive medical management for the control of type 2 diabetes, hypertension, and hyperlipidemia: the Diabetes Surgery Study randomized clinical trial. *JAMA* 2013; 309:2240-9.

[69] Zhang N, Maffei A, Cerabona T, et al. Reduction in obesity-related comorbidities: is gastric bypass better than sleeve gastrectomy? *Surg Endosc* 2013; 27:1273-80.

[70] Anderson KM, Castelli WP, Levy D. Cholesterol and mortality. 30 years of follow-up from the Framingham study. *JAMA* 1987; 257:2176-80.
[71] Joshi AV, Day D, Lubowski TJ, Ambegaonkar A. Relationship between obesity and cardiovascular risk factors: findings from a multi-state screening project in the United States. *Curr Med Res Opin* 2005; 21:1755-61.
[72] Nguyen NT, Varela E, Sabio A, et al. Resolution of hyperlipidemia after laparoscopic Roux-en-Y gastric bypass. *J Am Coll Surg* 2006; 203:24-9.
[73] Ruiz-Tovar J, Oller I, Tomas A, et al. Midterm impact of sleeve gastrectomy, calibrated with a 50-Fr bougie, on weight loss, glucose hemostasis, lipid profiles and comorbidities in morbidly obese patients. *Am Surg* 2012;78:969-74.
[74] Redline S, Budhiraja R, Kapur V, et al. The scoring of respiratory events in sleep: reliability and validity. *J Clin Sleep Med* 2007; 3:169-200.
[75] Sarkhosh K, Switzer NJ, El-Hadi M, et al. The impact of bariatric surgery on obstructive sleep apnea: a systematic review. *Obes Surg* 2013; 23:414-23.
[76] Madalosso CA, Gurski RR, Callegari-Jacques SM, et al. The impact of gastric bypass on gastroesophageal reflux disease in patients with morbid obesity: a prospective study based on the Montreal Consensus. *Ann Surg* 2010; 251:244-8.
[77] de Jong JR, Besselink MG, van Ramshorst B, et al. Effects of adjustable gastric banding on gastroesophageal reflux and esophageal motility: a systematic review. *Obes Rev* 2010; 11:297-305.
[78] Chiu S, Birch DW, Shi X, et al. Effect of sleeve gastrectomy on gastroesophageal reflux disease: a systematic review. *Surg Obes Relat Dis* 2011; 7:510-5.
[79] Rosenthal RJ, International Sleeve Gastrectomy Expert Panel, Diaz AA, et al. International Sleeve Gastrectomy Expert Panel Consensus Statement: best practice guidelines based on experience of >12,000 cases. *Surg Obes Relat Dis* 2012; 8:8-19.
[80] Vrbikova J, Hainer V. Obesity and polycystic ovary syndrome. *Obes Facts* 2009; 2:26-35.
[81] Eid GM, Cottam DR, Velcu LM, et al. Effective treatment of polycystic ovarian syndrome with Roux-en-Y gastric bypass. *Surg Obes Relat Dis* 2005; 1:77-80.
[82] Escobar-Morreale HF, Botella-Carretero JI, Alvarez-Blasco F, et al. The polycystic ovary syndrome associated with morbid obesity may resolve after weight loss induced by bariatric surgery. *J Clin Endocrinol Metab* 2005; 90:6364-9.
[83] Raghavendra RS, Kini D. Benign, premalignant, and malignant lesions encountered in bariatric surgery. *JSLS* 2012; 16:360-72.
[84] Basen-Engquist K, Chang M. Obesity and cancer risk: recent review and evidence. *Curr Oncol Rep* 2011; 13:71-6.
[85] Bardou M, Barkun AN, Martel M. Obesity and colorectal cancer. *Gut* 2013; 62:933-47.
[86] Hafeez S, Ahmed MH. Bariatric surgery as potential treatment for nonalcoholic fatty liver disease: a future treatment by choice or by chance? *J Obes* 2013; 2013:839275.
[87] Day CP. Non-alcoholic fatty liver disease: current concepts and management strategies. *Clin Med* 2006; 6:19-25.
[88] Tai CM, Huang CK, Hwang JC, et al. Improvement of nonalcoholic fatty liver disease after bariatric surgery in morbidly obese Chinese patients. *Obes Surg* 2012; 22:1016-21.
[89] van Hout GC, Boekestein P, Fortuin FA, et al. Psychosocial functioning following bariatric surgery. *Obes Surg* 2006; 16:787-94.

[90] Mamplekou E, Komesidou V, Bissias Ch, et al. Psychological condition and quality of life in patients with morbid obesity before and after surgical weight loss. *Obes Surg* 2005; 15:1177-84.

[91] Green AE, Dymek-Valentine M, Pytluk S, et al. Psychosocial outcome of gastric bypass surgery for patients with and without binge eating. *Obes Surg* 2004; 14:975-85.

[92] Papageorgiou GM, Papakonstantinou A, Mamplekou E, et al. Pre- and postoperative psychological characteristics in morbidly obese patients. *Obes Surg* 2002; 12:534-9.

[93] van Hout GC, van Oudheusden I, van Heck GL. Psychological profile of the morbidly obese. *Obes Surg* 2004; 14:579-88.

[94] Guisado JA, Vaz FJ. Personality profiles of the morbidly obese after vertical banded gastroplasty. *Obes Surg* 2003; 13:394-8.

[95] Buddeberg-Fischer B, Klaghofer R, Sigrist S, Buddeberg C. Impact of psychosocial stress and symptoms on indication for bariatric surgery and outcome in morbidly obese patients. *Obes Surg* 2004; 14:361-9.

[96] Sarwer DB, Wadden TA, Moore RH, et al. Changes in quality of life and body image after gastric bypass surgery. *Surg Obes Relat Dis* 2010; 6:608-14.

[97] Hrabosky JI, Masheb RM, White MA, et al. A prospective study of body dissatisfaction and concerns in extremely obese gastric bypass patients: 6- and 12-month postoperative outcomes. *Obes Surg* 2006; 16:1615-21.

In: Bariatric Surgery
Editor: Mandy Chambers

ISBN: 978-1-63463-697-1

Chapter 4

Long Term Diabetes Outcomes After Bariatric Surgery

Richard W. Carroll[1,2], Jeremy D. Krebs[1,2] and Rinki Murphy[3]
[1]Centre for Endocrine, Diabetes, and Obesity Research,
Wellington Regional Hospital, Wellington, New Zealand
[2]Department of Medicine, University of Otago (Wellington Campus)
[3]Department of Medicine, University of Auckland, New Zealand

Abstract

Bariatric surgery was developed primarily as a therapy to induce weight loss. Indeed, those with type 2 diabetes were originally not considered surgical candidates due to the perceived high risk nature of surgery in these individuals. However, significant post-operative improvements in diabetes control were noted early in the history of bariatric surgery. Multiple retrospective and prospective studies have since supported this finding, including a number of high quality randomised trials. Variable definitions of diabetes outcomes are used within the published literature complicating comparative analysis. This chapter will review the published literature on glycaemic outcomes at least 12 months following bariatric surgery, and discuss the importance of a consistent set of definitions when reporting on diabetes outcomes.

Introduction

Bariatric surgery was developed to induce weight loss, and was not originally proposed as a treatment for type 2 diabetes. Indeed, the majority of bariatric surgeons considered a diagnosis of type 2 diabetes to be a contraindication to bariatric surgery, due to a perception of increased surgical risk. Nonetheless, early pioneers of bariatric surgery recognised the early and sustained glycaemic benefits that those with pre-operative type 2 diabetes appeared to gain from surgery. Whilst the mechanism of this effect remains to be completely clarified, the concept of a surgical procedure as an appropriate and effective therapy for type 2 diabetes has been accepted following the publication of an increasing number of studies reporting superior outcomes in those undergoing surgery when compared to optimal lifestyle and medical treatment. Thus, in 2011, the International Diabetes Federation published a position statement on the place of bariatric surgery in the treatment armoury for type 2 diabetes. [1] This concluded by acknowledging that bariatric surgery should be considered earlier in the management of obese persons with type 2 diabetes. In this chapter, we discuss a number of recent studies that have contributed to this opinion.

The published literature on diabetes outcomes following bariatric surgery is extensive, and the quality of study methodology is variable. For the purposes of this chapter, a systematic literature search was performed to capture all studies published up to mid-2014. Search terms included 'bariatric surgery', 'gastric banding', 'sleeve gastrectomy', 'gastric bypass' 'biliopancreatic diversion', and 'diabetes'. In addition, the reference lists in included studies along with recent review articles were screened for appropriate studies not detected by the search. [2] Studies of bariatric surgery versus a non-surgical group or alternative bariatric procedures, that reported glycaemic outcomes at least 12 months following surgery were selected for discussion. The design of each of these studies varies, and the list includes prospective randomised controlled studies, and prospective and retrospective case controlled studies. Additionally, a number of meta-analyses including data from smaller, uncontrolled studies are discussed. A summary of the included studies is presented in table 1.

Definition of Diabetes Outcome

The state of diabetes following bariatric surgery and the definition of this has been highly controversial. A number of descriptions of glycaemic outcome to encompass varying degrees of diabetes resolution are utilised within the bariatric surgery literature. However, use of terms such as 'cure', 'resolved' or 'remission' in this context are controversial for a number of reasons. Most importantly, fasting glucose concentrations in the population are a continuous variable and the diagnosis of diabetes itself is based on a somewhat arbitrary threshold above which there is an increased risk of microvascular complications. It is not yet known whether these thresholds remain true in a post-bariatric surgery population, and consequently diagnostic criteria validated for a non-surgical population may be misleading when applied to those who have undergone bariatric surgery. Secondly, the concept of "glycaemic memory" is well established, and relates to the latent effect that periods of hyperglycaemia may have on outcomes later life, irrespective of changes in glycaemic control in the intervening period. [3] The UKPDS trial illustrated this concept most vividly. Participants randomised to the intensive treatment arm of the study had significantly improved glycaemic control over the 13 years of the study in comparison to those receiving standard treatment. [4] Participants were subsequently followed up 10 years after the completion of the study. Over this 10 year period glycaemic control, as measured using HbA1c, became comparable in the two groups. Despite this those who had been initially randomised to the intensive therapy arm maintained significantly lower rates of microvascular complications and cardiovascular mortality. This strongly argues that the period of early improved glycaemic control had a long term benefit on cardiovascular disease.

Table 1. Summary of discussed studies. Diabetes outcomes reported by each included study are presented, although the reader should note the different definitions utilized

Study	Intervention 1	Intervention 2	Duration of follow up	Study design	Definition of diabetes outcome	Diabetes at baseline (%)		Diabetes outcome at study end (%) based on study specific definition[1]	
						Intervention 1	Intervention 2	Intervention 1	Intervention 2
Hofso [6]	Gastric bypass	Lifestyle	12 months	Prospective case control	Complete = FG <5.6 mmol/L, and 2HrG of <7.8 mmol/L, and HbA1c of < 6.2% (44 mmol/mol) in the absence of glucose lowering therapy. Partial = FG <7.0 mmol/L, and 2HrG<11.1 mmol/L, and HbA1c < 6.5% (47 mmol/mol).	26	29	55 (70) [2]	0 (33)
Ikramuddin [7]	Gastric bypass	Lifestyle	12 months	Randomised	HbA1c <7% (53 mmol/L)	100	100	75	32
Kashyap et [12]	Gastric bypass/ Sleeve gastrectomy	Medical therapy	12 months	Randomised	HbA1c <6.0% (42 mmol/mol)	100	100	44 / 23	6
Lee [9]	Gastric bypass	Sleeve gastrectomy	12 months	Randomised	FG <126 mg/dl (7.0 mmol/L) and HbA1c of <6.5% (47 mmol/mol) in the absence of glucose lowering medications	100	100	93	47

[1] Figures in parentheses represent number achieving partial/incomplete control as per study specific definitions, unless otherwise indicated

[2] Diabetes outcome inclusive of participants who achieved either complete or partial remission.

Table 1. (Continued)

Study	Intervention 1	Intervention 2	Duration of follow up	Study design	Definition of diabetes outcome	Diabetes at baseline (%)		Diabetes outcome at study end (%) based on study specific definition[3]	
						Intervention 1	Intervention 2	Intervention 1	Intervention 2
Schauer [10]	Gastric bypass/ sleeve gastrectomy	Lifestyle	12 months	Randomised	HbA1c <42 mmol/mol with or without the use of diabetes medications	100	100	42 / 37[4]	12
Scopinaro [11]	Biliopancreatic diversion	Medical therapy	12 months	Prospective historical case control	FG <126mg/dl (7.0 mmol/L) and HbA1c <6.0% (42 mmol/mol) in the absence of glucose lowering medications	100	100	30 (83[5])	0
Serrot [8]	Gastric bypass	Medical therapy	12 months	Retrospective case control	HbA1c <5.7% (39 mmol/mol) in the absence of glucose lowering medications for remission, HbA1c <6.5% (47 mmol/mol) in the absence of glucose lowering medications for control	100	100	24 / 41	NR
Vidal [11]	Gastric bypass	Sleeve gastrectomy	12 months	Prospective comparison	FG <126 mg/dl (7.0 mmol/L), and HbA1c 3.4-5.5% (14-36 mmol/mol) in the absence of glucose lowering medications	100	100	85	85

[3] Figures in parentheses represent number achieving partial/incomplete control as per study specific definitions, unless otherwise indicated
[4] 5/18 in SG arm reported as achieving diabetes remission remained on diabetes medications, whilst none of those in remissionin RYGB arm did
[5] Inclusive of participants who were deemed to have achieved diabetes control defined as an HbA1c <7.0% (53 mmol/mol) in the absence of glucose lowering medication

Study	Intervention 1	Intervention 2	Duration of follow up	Study design	Definition of diabetes outcome	Diabetes at baseline (%)		Diabetes outcome at study end (%) based on study specific definition[6]	
						Intervention 1	Intervention 2	Intervention 1	Intervention 2
Adams [15]	Gastric bypass	Referred for but did not undergo surgery/ Population control	24 months	Prospective comparison	Hba1c and fasting glucose within the normal reference range	NR	NR	75	7 / 6
Dixon [16]	Laparoscopic adjustable gastric band	Lifestyle	24 months	Randomised	FG <126 mg/dl (7.0 mmol/L) and Hba1c <6.2% (44 mmol/mol) in the absence of glucose lowering therapy	100	100	73	23[7]
Kashyap [12]	Gastric bypass / Sleeve gastrectomy	Medical therapy	24 months	Randomised	HbA1c <6.0% (42 mmol/mol)	100	100	33 / 11	6
Leslie [14]	Gastric bypass	Medical therapy	24 months	Retrospective case control	Composite end point of ADA defined treatment goals (HbA1c<7.0% (53 mmol/mol), LDL<100mg/dl, SBP<130mmHg)	100	100	38	17
Mingrone [18]	Gastric bypass/ biliopancreatic diversion	Medical/ Lifestyle	24 months	Randomised	FG < 100 mg/dl (5.6 mmol/L) and HbA1c level < 6.5% (45 mmol/mol) for at least 1 year without active pharmacologic therapy	100	100	75 / 95	0

[6] Figures in parentheses represent number achieving partial/incomplete control as per study specific definitions, unless otherwise indicated

[7] Assuming that all those not available for follow up at study end (n=4) achieved diabetes remission. Diabetes remission achieved by 11% if each of these participants failed to achieved diabetes remission

Table 1. (Continued)

Study	Intervention 1	Intervention 2	Duration of follow up	Study design	Definition of diabetes outcome	Diabetes at baseline (%)		Diabetes outcome at study end (%) based on study specific definition[8]	
						Intervention 1	Intervention 2	Intervention 1	Intervention 2
Sjostrom [17]	Bariatric surgery[9]	Medical/Lifestyle[10]	24 months	Prospective case control	FG < 7.0 mmol/L or the use of glucose lowering medication	100	100	72	21
Pournaras et [22]	Gastric bypass	Gastric band	36 months	Prospective comparison	FG <7.0 mmol/L and 2hrG <11.1 mmol/L and HbA1c <42 mmol/mol in the absence of glucose lowering medication for > 3 months	100	100	72	17
Schauer [23][11]	Gastric bypass/ sleeve gastrectomy	Lifestyle	36 months	Randomised	HbA1c <42 mmol/mol with or without the use of diabetes medications	100	100	38 / 24	5
Pinheiro [21]	Gastric bypass [12]	Gastric bypass [13]	48 months	Randomised	Normal range glucose levels in the absence of glucose lowering medication	100	100	93	58

[8] Figures in parentheses represent number achieving partial/incomplete control as per study specific definitions, unless otherwise indicated
[9] Inclusive of gastric banding, sleeve gastrectomy, and gastric bypass
[10] Medical/lifestyle arm was not standardised
[11] Further follow up of participants reported earlier by Schauer et al. 91% of participants available for this further analysis
[12] Biliary limb of 50cm, Roux limb of 150cm
[13] Biliary limb of 100cm, Roux limb of 250cm

Study	Intervention 1	Intervention 2	Duration of follow up	Study design	Definition of diabetes outcome	Diabetes at baseline (%)		Diabetes outcome at study end (%) based on study specific definition[14]	
						Intervention 1	Intervention 2	Intervention 1	Intervention 2
Pontiroli [20]	Laparoscopic adjustable gastric band	Offered but declined laparoscopic adjustable gastric band	48 months	Prospective case control	FG < 6.1 mmol/L, and 2hrG <7.8 mmol/L in the absence of glucose lowering medications[15]	100	100	45	4
Adams [15]	Gastric bypass	Referred for, but did not undergo surgery/ Population control	72 months	Prospective case control	Hba1c and fasting glucose within the normal reference range	NR	NR	62	8 / 6
Iaconelli [19]	Biliopancreatic diversion	Medical therapy	120 months	Prospective case control	Not specified – implied that contemporary criteria for the diagnosis of diabetes used	100	100	100	45[16]
Sjostrom [17]	Bariatric surgery[17]	Medical/Lifestyle[18]	120 months	Prospective case control	FG < 7.0 mmol/L or the use of glucose lowering medication	100	100	36	13

[14] Figures in parentheses represent number achieving partial/incomplete control as per study specific definitions, unless otherwise indicated.

[15] Definition not defined in manuscript – implication that remission is defined by fasting and 2 hour OGTT glucose levels below contemporary diagnostic thresholds for dysglycaemia.

[16] Remission rate at 12 months – 120 month figure not provided, although mean HbA1c at that stage was 62 mmol/mol.

[17] Inclusive of gastric banding, sleeve gastrectomy, and gastric bypass.

[18] Medical/lifestyle arm was not standardized.

Therefore it cannot be assumed that if a person with diabetes has "normal" glucose metabolism following bariatric surgery, that their risk of micro and macro vascular disease is the same as a person who has never had a diagnosis of diabetes. It is highly plausible, and indeed worthy of study, that the glucose burden pre bariatric surgery confers an increased risk of micro and macrovascular disease later in life, even if normal glucose levels are restored following surgery. Furthermore, progressive decline in pancreatic beta cell function over time is characteristic of type 2 diabetes and it is unknown whether bariatric surgery alters this process. Thirdly, use of the term "cure" for a chronic disease mediated predominantly by lifestyle may not be helpful in encouraging longer term compliance to favourable dietary and exercise strategies. Regardless of these caveats, a better understanding of glycaemic outcomes following bariatric surgery is important for pre-operative patient counselling as to the likely glycaemic benefits from the procedure.

In the absence of definitive evidence addressing each of the issues above, the literature reporting diabetes outcomes following bariatric surgery is notable for the degree of variability with which diabetes remission is defined. This is confusing, and has possibly contributed to the delays seen for bariatric surgery to be accepted as an appropriate therapeutic option in the management of obese persons with type 2 diabetes. An agreed set of definitions of diabetes outcomes would ideally be used when reporting on bariatric surgery outcomes, and thus the American Diabetes Association (ADA) released a consensus statement in 2009 providing recommendations on the definition of glycaemic outcomes post bariatric surgery.[5] This suggested the use of the terms "partial remission" (HbA1C<6.5% (47 mmol/L), fasting glucose 100-125 mg/dl (5.6 – 6.9 mmol/L)), and "complete remission" (HbA1c "in the normal range", fasting glucose <100mg/dl (5.6 mmol/L)) provided that each of these assessments were persistent for at least 1 year duration, and in the absence of active pharmacologic therapy or ongoing procedures. Additionally, the ADA defined prolonged remission as the thresholds required for satisfaction of complete remission, maintained for at least 5 years. The definition of diabetes outcomes used by each study discussed below is variable, and the reader is therefore advised to consider the effect the chosen definition may have on outcome interpretation. Furthermore, comparison of bariatric surgery with non-surgical intensive medical management can only rely on achievement of similar glycaemic targets rather than diabetes remission as defined by achieving such glycaemic targets in the absence of glucose lowering therapy.

Review of Diabetes Outcomes Following Bariatric Procedures

The literature reporting on diabetes outcomes following bariatric surgery is extensive and ranges from small case series through to high quality randomised controlled studies. A number of excellent meta-analyses have attempted to address this diversity of study quality, and some of these publications are discussed later in this chapter. Here, we selected only those studies that included a comparison or control group, either an alternative bariatric procedure or lifestyle/medical therapies, and reported on outcomes at 12 months or beyond.

Studies Reporting Diabetes Outcomes at 12 Months

Gastric Bypass Versus Lifestyle/Medical Therapy

Three studies were identified reporting diabetes outcomes at 12 months following gastric bypass.[6-8] Diabetes control was achieved by 41-75% of those in the gastric bypass arm in these studies. The variability is likely due to differences in the definitions utilised to define diabetes outcomes in each study and in the baseline characteristics of the participants. The study by Ikramuddin and colleagues defined only diabetes control and accepted a higher HbA1c threshold (<7.0% (53 mmol/mol)) than the other two studies; thus, this study reported the highest rates of diabetes control. The studies by Hofso and Serrot both reported diabetes remission, requiring absence of glucose lowering medications, and control defined by a lower HbA1c level, a higher mean age of participant in the surgical arm (56 vs 42 years), and a higher HbA1c at baseline (8.2 vs 7.1% (66 vs 54 mmol/mol)).

Hofso and colleagues performed a comparison study of gastric bypass versus a lifestyle based intervention in 146 morbidly obese adults (mean BMI 45.6 kg/m2) and reported outcomes at 12 months.[6] The study was not randomised as the study authors considered this to be unethical on the basis of clear local guidelines on selecting bariatric interventions for obese patients. Those in the gastric bypass arm of the study received a low calorie diet for 3 to 6 weeks prior to surgery, and were seen by a dietitian in group sessions every 3 months during the study period. The lifestyle intervention in this study was significant; each participant in this arm was referred to a specialist inpatient weight loss centre and had four stays within the centre during the 12 month study period. Each admission was for between 1 and 4 weeks. Participants received numerous interventions during each stay including input from a medical doctor, a nurse, a physiotherapist, and a specialist trained nurse. Physical activity was increased, and all participants were provided with education on a healthy diet, which they were encouraged to follow. Group sessions focused on the psychosocial and emotional aspects of obesity and weight loss. Weight loss drugs were not used. Phone contact was maintained fortnightly while participants were away from the weight loss centre. In addition to fasting bloods, a 75g 2 hour oral glucose tolerance test was used to define both diabetes at study entry and diabetes outcomes. 26% and 29% of participants in the gastric bypass and lifestyle intervention arms respectively had type 2 diabetes at baseline. Diabetes remission was defined as a fasting glucose <5.6 mmol/L, and a 2 hour glucose of <7.8 mmol/L, and an HbA1c of < 6.2% (44 mmol/mol) in the absence of glucose lowering therapy. In addition, the study authors defined partial diabetes remission as glucose levels below the diagnostic thresholds at baseline (<7.0 and 11.1 mmol/L for fasting and 2 hour glucose respectively) and an HbA1c < 6.5% (47 mmol/mol) without the use of glucose lowering therapy.

The study authors elected to report diabetes remission rates at 12 months, including participants who had achieved either complete or partial remission. Thus, the overall diabetes remission rate by this criteria was significantly greater in the gastric bypass arm versus those in the lifestyle intervention arm (70 vs 33%, OR 4.7 (1.2–18.4). However, none of the participants in the lifestyle intervention arm achieved complete diabetes remission, whilst 11 out of the 14 participants (55% of those with type 2 diabetes at baseline) achieved complete diabetes remission at 12 months follow up.

Ikramuddin and colleagues performed a 12 month randomised study of intensive medical management versus intensive medical management plus Roux-en-Y gastric bypass.[7] 120 obese participants (BMI 30-39 kg/m2) with type 2 diabetes were recruited, and a primary composite outcome incorporating achievement of diabetes, blood pressure and lipid control targets was reported. Intensive medical management included a reduced energy diet for all participants with the aim of weight loss in the order of 1-2 pounds per week. Increased physical activity was encouraged, and each participant had regular face to face contact with a study interventionist to discuss behavioural and social issues around weight loss. Orlistat, and Sibutramine prior to withdrawal from the US market, were available for use by those in the lifestyle arm if agreed weight loss targets were not met. The contemporary American Diabetes Association guidelines for the management of type 2 diabetes were followed for the medical management of each participant in the study. 75% of those randomised to gastric bypass achieved diabetes control (defined solely as an HbA1c of <7% (53 mmol/L)) at 12 months versus 32% of those randomised to intensive medical management only (OR, 6.0; 95% CI, 2.6-13.9). Whilst the primary composite outcome was achieved in 49% (versus 19%) of those undergoing gastric bypass, there was no difference between the two arms when blood pressure and lipid outcomes were assessed as independent outcomes.

Serrot and colleagues performed a retrospective case control study of obese (BMI 30-35 kg/m2) participants with type 2 diabetes who had undergone gastric bypass in their institution versus a control group (BMI matched persons with type 2 diabetes from a primary care database).[8] Of nearly 3000 gastric bypass procedures performed over an 8 year period, 20% had preoperative type 2 diabetes and of these, 17 participants had a BMI of 30-35 kg/m2. Each surgical participant was matched with one control subject. Diabetes remission was defined as an HbA1c <5.7% (39 mmol/mol) in the absence of glucose lowering medications, whilst diabetes control was defined as an HbA1c <6.5% (47 mmol/mol) in the absence of glucose lowering medications. At the 12 month follow up assessment 4/17 (24%) of surgical participants had achieved diabetes remission and a further 7 (41%) of participants had achieved diabetes control. Classification outcomes in the control group were not reported. The mean HbA1c in those who had undergone surgery fell from a baseline level of 8.2% ((66 mmol/mol) ± 2.0%) to 6.1% ((43 mmol/mol) ± 2.7%), but did not change significantly in the control group ((7.0 (53 mmol/mol) ± 0.7% to 7.1 (54 mmol/mol) ± 1.8%).

Gastric Bypass versus Sleeve Gastrectomy

Two randomised controlled studies and one prospective non-randomised study reported outcomes at 12 months following either gastric bypass or sleeve gastrectomy, with 2 of these studies including a lifestyle/medical arm.[9-11] In addition, a further randomised controlled study primarily reporting on 24 month outcomes, presented 12 month outcomes.[12] Whilst each study used stringent criteria for diabetes remission/control, it should be noted that participants in the study by Lee and colleagues demonstrating superior efficacy of GBP compared to SG, these participants were Taiwanese and had significantly lower BMI at baseline versus those in the studies by Schauer and Vidal which both showed similar efficacy of GBP compared to SG. The apparent marked increase in surgical participants achieving diabetes remission in the study by Vidal when compared to those in the study by Schauer (85% versus 40%) is of interest. Despite a similar age at surgery (mean approximately 48 years), participants in the Schauer study were not as obese, had a longer pre-operative duration of diabetes, and a 4 fold higher pre-operative use of insulin. This may indicate less beta cell reserve, and thus reduced likelihood of resolution of diabetes even with substantive weight loss and improved insulin sensitivity.

Lee and colleagues reported 12 month diabetes outcomes following randomisation to gastric bypass or sleeve gastrectomy in 60 overweight (BMI 25-35 kg/m2) Taiwanese participants with sub-optimally controlled type 2 diabetes.[9] Diabetes remission was defined as a fasting glucose of <126 mg/dl (7.0 mmol/L) and HbA1c of <6.5% (47 mmol/mol) and the absence of diabetes medications. Participants were assessed by an extensive multidisciplinary team prior to surgery but the study does not report on medical interventions used in the post-operative period. 93% of those randomised to gastric bypass achieved diabetes remission at 12 months versus 47% of those who had undergone sleeve gastrectomy.

Schauer and colleagues first reported on diabetes outcomes of overweight and obese American participants (BMI 27-43 kg/m2) and type 2 diabetes at 12 months of follow up.[10] 150 participants were recruited and randomised in equal numbers to one of 3 interventional arms (intensive medical therapy, gastric bypass plus intensive medical management, and sleeve gastrectomy plus intensive medical management). Diabetes control/remission, defined as an HbA1c <42 mmol/mol with or without the use of diabetes medications, was achieved by 12% of those randomised to medical therapy only, 42% of those randomised to the gastric bypass arm, and 37% of those randomised to the sleeve gastrectomy arm. The definition of diabetes remission utilised for this study was clearly limited by the acceptance of an HbA1c < 42 mmol/mol as evidence for remission even in the context of ongoing diabetes medication use. It could be argued that those who required ongoing glucose lowering therapy should be defined as being, at best, partial responders. However, all of those in the gastric bypass arm who achieved diabetes remission did so without the ongoing use of diabetes medications, whilst 28% of those in the sleeve gastrectomy arm who were reported as achieving diabetes remission continued to require glucose lowering therapy; all of those in the medical management alone arm who achieved the primary endpoint remained on glucose lowering therapy.

Vidal and colleagues performed a non-randomised prospective study comparing outcomes of severely obese (BMI >35kg/m2) participants with type 2 diabetes (n=91) who underwent either gastric bypass (n=52) or laparoscopic sleeve gastrectomy (n=39).[11] The groups were matched at baseline for duration, control, and treatment of diabetes. Diabetes remission was defined as a fasting glucose <126 mg/dl (7.0 mmol/L) and an HbA1c within the normal range (3.4-5.5% (14-37 mmol/mol)) in the absence of glucose lowering medications. At 12 months following surgery diabetes remission had been achieved by 84.6% of those who had undergone gastric bypass and 84.6% of those who had undergone laparoscopic sleeve gastrectomy. Interestingly, the study authors found no relationship between weight loss and diabetes remission, but did note a significant association between duration and severity (treatments required, HbA1c at baseline) of diabetes and diabetes remission.

Biliopancreatic Diversion versus Lifestyle/Medical Therapy

Scopinaro and colleagues performed a prospective, case controlled study of biliopancreatic diversion surgery versus medical management in overweight or obese persons (BMI 25-34.9 kg/m2) with type 2 diabetes.[13] Participants who underwent biliopancreatic diversion surgery had a mean age of 56 years and established diabetes (mean duration of diabetes = 11 years, mean HbA1c at baseline = 78 mmol/mol, 12/30 participants requiring insulin therapy at baseline). Controls were selected from an historical registry. The study authors defined 3 categories of diabetes outcomes. Diabetes remission was defined as a fasting glucose <126 mg/dl (7.0 mmol/L), and an HbA1c ≤6.0% (42 mmol/mol) without the use of glucose lowering medications; controlled diabetes was defined as an HbA1c ≤7.0% (53 mmol/mol) in the absence of glucose lowering medication; improved diabetes was defined as a >1% (10-11 mmol/mol) reduction in Hba1c levels when compared to baseline. No participants in the historical control group achieved diabetes remission or diabetes control during 1 year of treatment (mean HbA1c at baseline = 8.8% (73 mmol/mol)). Whilst two thirds of participants required an increase in their medication doses during this 12 month period, no participant was able to reduce medication doses. In contrast, diabetes remission was achieved by 30% of those who had undergone biliopancreatic diversion, and diabetes control by a further 53% (83% total). However, 5 participants (out of 12) who required insulin therapy at baseline remained on insulin therapy at 12 months following biliopancreatic surgery.

The relative low rate of diabetes remission following biliopancreatic diversion in this study, in contrast to very high rates more commonly reported following this procedure, may be explained by the baseline characteristics of the study cohort. Specifically, this was an older cohort than other studies discussed above (mean age = 56.4 years), and participants had both a longer duration of diabetes (mean = 11.2 years) and a higher Hba1c (mean = 9.6% (81 mmol/mol)) at baseline.

Studies Reporting on Outcomes from 12 to 24 Months

Gastric Bypass versus Lifestyle/Medical Therapy

Two study of gastric bypass versus lifestyle medical therapy were identified that reported on outcomes at 24 months.[14,15] The study by Adams and colleagues continued to follow up their cohort for a total of 72 months and is therefore discussed in the following section. Leslie and colleagues performed a retrospective case control study of outcomes following gastric bypass versus medical managements for obese persons with type 2 diabetes.[14] Rather than define diabetes outcomes using simply glycaemic markers, the study authors elected to use a composite end point of treatment goals as recommended by the American Diabetes Association for the management of type 2 diabetes (HbA1c <7.0% (53 mmol/mol), low-density lipoprotein <100mg/dl, systolic blood pressure <130mmHg). 152 and 115 participants who had undergone gastric bypass or medical therapy alone respectively were included in the analysis. The percentage of participants satisfying the ADA treatment goals who had undergone gastric bypass was 10.5% at baseline, increasing to 38.2% at 24 months follow up. A smaller, non-significant increase was noted in the medical therapy group (13.9% at baseline versus 17.4% at 24 months).

Laparoscopic Adjustable Gastric Band versus Lifestyle/Medical Therapy

One study was identified that reported on diabetes outcomes 24 months following laparoscopic adjustable gastric banding. Dixon and colleagues reported diabetes outcomes at 24 months on 60 obese participants (BMI 30-40 kg/m2, age range 20-60 years) with type 2 diabetes randomised to either laparoscopic adjustable gastric banding or an intensive lifestyle program without the use of bariatric surgery.[16] The lifestyle program was comprehensive and administered via a multidisciplinary team consisting of a physician, dietitian, and diabetes nurse via face to face meetings at 6 week intervals. A low energy diet with reduced saturated fats was prescribed along with increased exercise activity; very low calorie diets and/or weight loss pharmaceutical agents were also available for use. Diabetes remission was defined as a fasting glucose level of <126 mg/dl (7.0 mmol/L) and an Hba1c <6.2% (44 mmol/mol) in the absence of glucose lowering therapy, and was achieved by 73% of those who in the laparoscopic adjustable gastric band arm versus 11-23% (based on the assumption that diabetes remission was/was not achieved by 4 participants randomised to the lifestyle arm who did not complete the study). Furthermore, improvement in diabetes control was evident in those who underwent gastric banding with 26/30 participants not requiring glucose lowering therapy at study end (versus 2 at baseline).

The percentage of participants who achieved diabetes remission in the surgical arm of this study was high, and particularly notable given that the mean age at which participants underwent surgery (46.6 years), the mean HbA1c at baseline (7.8% (62 mmol/mol)), and a mean BMI at surgery (37.0 kg/m2) was comparable to baseline characteristics of cohorts in other studies discussed in this chapter following gastric bypass or biliopancreatic diversion surgery. However, only one participant in the surgical group used insulin therapy at baseline, and although duration of diabetes at surgery was not reported, the exclusion of participants with evidence of microvascular complications is likely to result in the selection of those with a more recent diagnosis of diabetes.

Bariatric Surgery versus Lifestyle/Medical Therapy

Three studies were identified that reported on outcomes in studies incorporating two or more bariatric surgery modalities.[12,17,18] The Swedish Obesity Study (SOS) reported on outcomes at 24 months in addition to those at 120 months and is thus discussed in the section below.[17] The studies by Kashyap and Mingrone both included a gastric bypass arm but reported markedly different diabetes outcomes at 24 months (33 versus 75% respectively). The authors used significantly different definitions of diabetes outcomes that could potentially result in discordant outcomes. However, whilst Kashyap elected to simply use HbA1c, Mingrone utilised seemingly more stringent criteria including a fasting glucose and HbA1c threshold, and the absence of glucose lowering medication. It should be noted though that Mingrone accepted an HbA1c of <6.5% (47 mmol/mol) as evidence of diabetes remission. The discordance between these studies is also not easily explained by differing baseline characteristics; whilst the two cohorts undergoing gastric bypass were of similar ages at operation (mean = 47.9 years and 43.9 years for the Kashyap and Mingrone studies respectively), and had a similar duration and control of diabetes at baseline (7.4/6.0 years, 9.0%(75 mmol/mol)/8.5%(69 mmol/mol) respectively), participants in the Mingrone study had a significantly higher BMI (44.6 versus 36.1 kg/m2). Additionally, differences in the medical/lifestyle program, prescribed for those in the surgical arms alongside surgery, do not appear likely to be a factor in this anomaly. None of the medical/lifestyle arm of the Mingrone study achieved diabetes remission, in comparison to 6% of participants in the equivalent arm of the Kashyap study.

Kashyap and colleagues undertook a prospective randomised study of optimal medical therapy versus either gastric bypass or sleeve gastrectomy in 60 moderately obese (mean BMI =36.1 kg/m2) participants with type 2 diabetes at baseline.[12] All patients received intensive medical therapy as recommended by the American Diabetes Association, including dietary modifications, increased frequency of capillary glucose measurements, and the use of all available glucose lowering agents. In addition, each participant received nutritional counselling by a study dietitian and underwent a psychological assessment, in part to assess suitability for bariatric surgery. Participants were then randomly allocated to either ongoing medical therapy alone, gastric bypass surgery, or sleeve gastrectomy. Diabetes remission was defined as an HbA1c of less than 42 mmol/mol (6.0%). 44% and 26% of those who had undergone gastric bypass and sleeve gastrectomy respectively had an HbA1c of <6.0% (42 mmol/mol) at 12 months follow up, compared with 6% of those who had received medical therapy alone. However, a reduction in the number of participants satisfying criteria for diabetes control at 24 months was evident (33, 11, and 6% for gastric bypass, sleeve gastrectomy, and medical therapy respectively).

Mingrone and colleagues performed a single centre randomised controlled study of gastric bypass versus biliopancreatic diversion versus medical/lifestyle therapy only.[18] 60 participants (age 30-60, BMI >35 kg/m2) were recruited, each of whom had had type 2 diabetes for at least 5 years and had a current HbA1c of >7.0% (53 mmol/mol). Each participant had visits with a multidisciplinary team (including a diabetologist, dietitian, and study nurse) at baseline and then 1, 3, 6, 9, 12 and 24 months following commencement of the intervention. A low-fat, high fibre diet and ≥30 minutes of brisk walking every day was prescribed to those in the medical arm and diabetes medications were adjusted based on regular HbA1c measurements. In keeping with the definition suggested by the American Diabetes Association, diabetes remission was defined as a fasting plasma glucose level < 100 mg/dl (5.6 mmol/L) and an HbA1c level < 6.5% (45 mmol/mol) for at least 1 year without active pharmacologic therapy. Diabetes remission was achieved by 95% of those in the biliopancreatic diversion arm, 75% of those in the gastric bypass arm, and none of those in the medical arm. Biliopancreatic diversion and gastric bypass were associated with an odds ratio of diabetes remission of at least 9.5 (95% CI, 2.54 to 35.51; P<0.001) and 7.5 (95% CI 1.97 to 28.61; P<0.001) respectively when compared with medical therapy alone.

As noted earlier, the 95% diabetes remission rate in the biliopancreatic diversion arm of the above study by Mingrone and colleagues is significantly higher than the 30% at 12 months seen in the study by Scopinaro discussed in the section above. Again, this is likely to be explained by the older age at surgery, and longer duration of diabetes of participants in the Scopinaro study.

Studies Reporting on Outcomes beyond 2 Years

Bariatric Surgery versus Lifestyle/Medical Therapy

Adams and colleagues performed a prospective study recruiting obese adults (BMI>35kg/m2) who underwent gastric bypass surgery over a 10 year period (n=418).[15] 2 control groups were included, the first of which included participants who had sought but not undergone gastric bypass surgery (n=417), and a second group comprised of obese adults selected from a regional registry (n=321). An explanation as to why each of the participants in the first control group had not undergone gastric bypass was not provided in the manuscript. The prevalence of diabetes within each group at baseline was not presented, although the mean HbA1c was 42 mmol/mol or less in each group. Diabetes at baseline was defined as a fasting glucose of >126mg/dl (7.0 mmol/l), and/or an HbA1c of >6.5% (47 mmol/mol), and/or the use of glucose lowering medications, whilst remission of diabetes was defined as an Hba1c and fasting glucose within the normal reference range (absolute figures not provided) in the absence of ongoing glucose lowering therapy. Using these definitions, diabetes remission was achieved by 75% (95% CI, 63%-87%) and 62% (95% CI, 49%-75%) at 2 and 6 years post-surgery respectively in the gastric bypass group. Diabetes remission rates at 6 years were significantly lower in those who had either sought gastric bypass but not undergone surgery (8%; 95%CI,0%-16%, OR, 16.5 versus gastric bypass) and population controls (6%; 95% CI, 0%-13%, OR, 21.5). The study authors also noted a significantly lower incidence of new diagnoses of diabetes during 6 year follow up in the gastric bypass group (2%; 95% CI, 0%-4%) in comparison to those in the first control group (17%; 95% CI 10%-24%, OR 0.11 favouring gastric bypass; 95% CI 0.04- 0.34) and those in the population control group (15%; 95% CI 9%- 21%, OR 0.21 favouring gastric bypass; 95% CI, 0.06-0.67).

Iaconelli and colleagues performed a prospective case controlled study of conventional lifestyle and medical therapy versus biliopancreatic diversion in obese participants with type 2 diabetes.[19] Diabetes outcomes were reported at 10 years. The study authors note the initial study design of a randomised controlled trial was declined by their ethics regulatory committee partly on the basis of the required long duration of follow up. Instead the study team enrolled 110 obese participants with type 2 diabetes and initiated a 3 month run-in intervention comprising dietary optimisation. At the end of the run-in period, participants who met the inclusion criteria for the study (age 25-60 years, BMI >35 kg/m2, and a residual diagnosis of type 2 diabetes on the basis of standard critieria, n=50) were offered either conventional lifestyle and medical therapy alone, or conventional therapy plus biliopancreatic diversion surgery (n=28 and 22 respectively). Conventional therapy included dietary, exercise and medication optimisation as per current American Diabetes Association guidelines. Diabetes remission was actually a secondary endpoint in the study, with the authors choosing instead change in the glomerular filtration rate from baseline to study end as their primary end point. The authors did not specify the definition used for diabetes remission in the study, although it is implied that diagnostic thresholds commonly used at the initiation of the study (fasting glucose >7.0 mmol/L (on 2 occasions) and/or a 2 hour glucose > 11.1 mmol/L following a 75g oral glucose tolerance test) were utilised to assess diabetes outcome. The manuscript provides no information on whether ongoing use of glucose lowering therapy was accounted for. Allowing for these limitations, diabetes remission was achieved by 100% of participants at 12 months by those who had undergone biliopancreatic diversion surgery; the authors noted that none of these participants redeveloped diabetes during the remainder of follow up to 10 years. The mean HbA1c at 10 years in the conventional treatment and biliopancreatic diversion surgery arms was 7.8% (62 mmol/mol) and 4.9% (30 mmol/mol) respectively.

Pontiroli and colleagues performed a prospective case controlled study of outcomes following laparoscopic adjustable gastric banding versus optimisation of lifestyle and medical therapies.[20] The study investigators recruited 122 sequential patients (age range 18-66) referred for the management of obesity, who met contemporary criteria for bariatric surgery (BMI > 40 kg/m2, or BMI > 35 kg/m2 in the presence of obesity related co-morbidities). The absence or presence of type 2 diabetes was clarified through an oral glucose tolerance test based on standard diagnostic criteria. The participants were then followed within two intervention studies; the primary intervention study assessed the effect of laparoscopic adjustable gastric banding on the prevention of type 2 diabetes, whilst the secondary intervention study assessed the effect on those with established type 2 diabetes. Thus, 37 participants with established type 2 diabetes were enrolled in the secondary intervention section of the study. Each of these participants was offered laparoscopic adjustable gastric banding; 17 consented to surgery with the remainder wishing to utilise lifestyle/medical options. The applied definition of diabetes remission was not specifically provided in the published manuscript, although it is implied that contemporary diagnostic criteria for the diagnosis of thresholds of dysglycaemia were utilised. Thus, diabetes remission would be diagnosed on the basis of a fasting glucose level <6.1 mmol/L, and a 2 hour post glucose level of <7.8 mmol/L (presumably also in the absence of glucose lowering medications). HbA1c measurements were recorded but are not specifically reported in the context of diabetes remission. Using this definition, diabetes remission was achieved by 45% at 4 years by those who had undergone laparoscopic adjustable gastric banding, and 4% of those who had declined surgery. Of note, none of those who had undergone laparoscopic adjustable gastric banding as a part of the primary prevention component of the study developed diabetes during the 4 years of follow up, whilst 17% of those who declined surgery did so.

Studies Comparing Different Forms of Bariatric Surgery

Pinheiro and colleagues performed a randomised study of two types of Roux-en-Y gastric bypass in 105 participants with type 2 diabetes and severe obesity (BMI >50kg/m2).[21] The diagnosis of diabetes and diabetes outcomes was defined on the basis of diagnostic thresholds. The primary intent of the study was to assess the varying effect of the resulting length of both the biliary and Roux limb of the gastric bypass. In group 1, the biliary and Roux limbs were 50 and 150 cm respectively, whilst in group 2 the biliary and Roux limbs were 100 and 250cm respectively (so called long-long limb Roux-en-Y gastric bypass). At 48 months follow up, diabetes control (glycaemic markers below diabetes diagnostic thresholds in the absence of glucose lowering medication) was achieved in 58% of those in group 1 and 93% of those in group 2. A statistically higher proportion of participants in group 2 had improvement of dyslipidaemia, whilst there was no difference in the improvement in hypertension seen.

Pournaras et al performed a prospective comparison study of gastric bypass (n=22) versus gastric banding (n=12) in severely obese participants with type 2 diabetes.[22] The study design allowed for an assessment of diabetes outcomes, along with exploration of the mechanism underlying the expected improvements in diabetes control. The study investigators defined diabetes remission based on contemporary diagnostic thresholds; a fasting plasma glucose <7 mmol/L in the absence of medical treatment for at least 3 days, and a 2-hour plasma glucose <11.1 mmol/L following an oral glucose tolerance test (OGTT). In addition, an HbA1c <6.0% (42 mmol/mol) after 3 months without the use of glucose lowering medication was required. Participants had established diabetes at baseline with a mean duration of diabetes of >5 years; 55% of those who underwent gastric bypass and 30% of those who underwent gastric banding required insulin therapy prior to surgery. 68% of those in the gastric bypass arm had achieved diabetes remission at 12 months of follow up versus none in the gastric banding arm despite similar weight loss (20-25% body weight) at that assessment. At 36 months follow up, the percentage of those in diabetes remission had increased to 72% and 17% for gastric bypass and gastric banding respectively.

Following publication of diabetes outcome results after bariatric surgery at 12 months,[10] Schauer and colleagues performed a further analysis of follow up outcomes at 36 months.[23] 137 (91%) of the original 150 randomised participants (randomised in equal numbers to intensive medical therapy, gastric bypass plus intensive medical therapy, and sleeve gastrectomy plus intensive medical therapy) were evaluated. As in the original study, diabetes remission was defined as an HbA1c of <42 mmol/mol with or without the use of diabetes medications, and was achieved by 38% and 24% of those who had undergone gastric bypass and sleeve gastrectomy respectively (versus 5% of those randomised to intensive medical therapy alone). Glycaemic relapse (defined as satisfying criteria for diabetes remission at 12 months but not at 36 months) was seen in 80% of participants in the medical therapy group, 24% of those who had undergone gastric bypass group, and 50% of those who had undergone sleeve gastrectomy. Decrease in BMI following surgery (odds ratio, 1.33 for every 1 unit (mg/m2); 95% CI, 1.15 to 1.56; P<0.001) and the pre-surgical duration of type 2 diabetes (duration <8 versus >8 years; odds ratio, 3.3; 95% CI, 1.2 to 9.1; P = 0.02) were the only two predictors of diabetes outcome following either bariatric surgery.

The Swedish Obese Subjects Study (SOS study) was a very large prospective non-randomised study performed in Sweden between 1987 and 2000.[17] Following a large scale national recruitment drive, 4047 participants who met the study criteria (BMI >34 kg/m2 for men, BMI >38 kg/m2 for women, age 37-60 years) were recruited and offered either non-surgical or, if appropriate, surgical interventions. Surgery was performed at 25 national centres and included gastric banding, sleeve gastrectomy, and gastric bypass. Each participant who had chosen bariatric surgery was matched at the time of surgery to a participant who had elected medical therapy only (based on 18 variables including demographic, metabolic, psychosocial, and personality parameters). Medical and lifestyle therapies were not standardised for this trial. The intervention for both the surgically treated participant, and their match medical therapy only control, was considered to have commenced on the day of surgery.

Outcomes following 10 years of follow up were reported in 2004 and included data on 4047 participants with at least 2 years of follow up data available (all those enrolled in the SOS study) and 1703 participants who had 10 years of follow up data available. The study authors reported both diabetes incidence (compared with baseline) and diabetes outcomes. The majority of enrolled participants did not have type 2 diabetes at baseline, although the study authors were still able to report on approximately 200 participants who did and had follow up data extending to 10 years. The criteria used to define both disease and disease outcome were the same, and were reflective of contemporary diabetes diagnostic thresholds. Thus, diabetes remission was defined as a fasting glucose of <7.0 mmol/L (126 mg/dl) in the absence of glucose lowering medications.

590/4047 and 202/4047 participants had type 2 diabetes at baseline and 2 or 10 years of follow up data available respectively. Of those with 2 years of follow up data, 246/342 (72%) of surgical participants and 52/248 (21%) of control participants had achieved diabetes remission (Odds ratio 8.42 95%CI 5.68-12.5). Over the same period, 8% of control participants who did not have diabetes at baseline (n=1402) developed type 2 diabetes, compared to 1% of those who had undergone bariatric surgery (n=1489). Of those with 10 years of follow up data, 42/118 (36%) of surgical participants and 11/84 (13%) of control subjects had achieved diabetes remission (Odds ratio 3.45 95%CI 1.64-7.28). As expected the incidence of new diabetes in those who did not have type 2 diabetes at baseline, had increased further at 10 years such that 24% and 7% of control and surgical participants respectively had developed diabetes.

Recently, the SOS study authors have reported on further long term outcomes at greater than 15 years.[31] These data provide further evidence that bariatric surgery has a favourable and durable effect on obesity and the risk of developing type 2 diabetes or related complications. Surgery reduced the risk of developing type 2 diabetes by 78% at 15 years, and reduced overall mortality by 29% (HR=0.71, 95%CI 0.54-0.92) at 16 years of follow up. Bariatric surgery was associated with a 53% reduction in the risk of fatal cardiovascular events (adjusted HR=0.47, 95%CI 0.29-0.78), and a 33% reduction in total cardiovascular events (HR=0.67, 95%CI 0.54-0.83) at up to 18 years of follow up. A reduction in the incidence of a new diagnosis of cancer following surgery (HR=0.67, 95%CI 0.53-0.85) was also demonstrated. On the basis that obesity is a known risk factor for cancer, this raises the possibility that intentional weight loss achieved by bariatric surgery may protect against this association although further research is required.

Meta-Analyses of Studies Reporting on Diabetes Outcomes Following Bariatric Surgery

A large number of meta-analyses using a diverse range of selection criteria have been published. The majority report on weight or short term outcomes only and are therefore beyond the scope of this chapter. The reader is directed towards meta-analyses performed by Lai, Maggard-Gibbons, and Gloy and colleagues which all included either studies discussed in the paragraphs above, or studies reporting on diabetes outcomes <12 months following surgery.[24-26] In addition, Parikh and colleagues have recently published a meta-analysis of 39 studies reporting on diabetes outcomes in subjects with a BMI <35kg/m2.[27]

The largest meta-analysis thus far published reporting outcomes of bariatric surgery (gastric banding, gastroplasty, RYGB and biliopancreatic diversion/duodenal switch (BD/DS)) included all studies published between 1990 and 2006, and updated a previous meta-analysis by the same group.[28,29] The meta-analysis included 621 studies, within which 103 arms specifically reported on diabetes outcomes (3188 subjects). All study designs were included, with each study was assigned a level of evidence. 22.3% of the cohort (30,160/135,246 subjects) had pre-operative diabetes. Weight loss across the whole cohort, expressed as excess body weight lost (EBWL%), was 48.98, 56.48, 63.25, and 73.72% at ≥ 2 year follow up for gastric banding, gastroplasty, RYGB, and BD/DS respectively, although the majority of subjects remained obese (Mean pre-operative BMI 47.86, mean post-operative BMI 33.89kg/m2). Weight loss assessed at ≥ 2 years exceeded that reported at shorter post-operative intervals for each modality. Weight loss in patients with pre-operative diabetes was similar with 67.1 and 58.01% EBWL at <2 or ≥ 2 year follow up respectively when all surgical modalities were included (67.10 and 64.7% for RYGB specifically). Analysis of the subjects with diabetes included in the meta-analysis revealed that resolution of diabetes (defined as cessation of diabetes medications and either normal fasting glucose (<100 mg/dl (5.5 mmol/L)) or an HbA1c < 6% (42 mmol/mol) across the whole cohort was 78.1% (80.27 and 74.59% at <2 and ≥ 2 year follow up respectively), whilst resolution or improvement (defined as a reduction in number or dose of diabetes medications, or an improvement in fasting glucose to between 100-125 mg/dl (5.5 - 6.9 mmol/L)) was seen in 86.61% (86.0 and 87.24% respectively). Further assessment based on surgical procedure revealed that resolution of diabetes was seen in 56.73% (54.99 and 58.29% at <2 and ≥ 2 year follow up respectively) following gastric banding, 79.74% (81.44 and 77.46%) following gastroplasty, 80.28% (81.60 and 70.90%) following RYGB, and 95.05% (94.0 and 95.85%) following BD/DS.

In addition the authors performed a sub-analysis on 12 studies that included only subjects with diabetes (n=963) and reported overall resolution of diabetes in 79.29% (81.81 and 62.08%), and resolution or improvement in 98.91% (98.56 and 100%). It should be noted however that data for ≥ 2 year follow up in studies that recruited only those with diabetes included only 48 subjects (31 who underwent RYGB and 17 who underwent gastric banding). Of those who underwent RYGB, 80.65% remained in remission from diabetes at ≥2 years whilst all patients had experienced at least improvement in glycaemic control. Less impressively, only 41% (7/17 subjects) who had undergone gastric banding remained in remission from diabetes at 2 years. Additionally, the definition of resolution or improvement of diabetes, or even the diagnosis of diabetes itself, varied significantly across the included studies. Overt diabetes was generally defined as an HbA1c of > 53 mmol/mol (7%) whilst most international organisations that accept HbA1c as a diagnostic tool currently suggest cut off values of between 45 and 50 mmol/mol, with a lower range reflective of less severe abnormalities in glucose homeostasis. Secondly, resolution of diabetes was confirmed in some studies on the basis of a measured fasting glucose without the requirement of either further testing or perhaps more robust HbA1c assessments. Improvements in diabetes control was also defined biochemically as a reduction of fasting glucose to between 5.5 -6.9 mmol/L irrespective of HbA1c. As the rationale behind glucose lowering in patients with diabetes is to prevent longer term micro and macrovascular complications, and HbA1c correlates best with the risk of these complications irrespective of day to day fluctuations in plasma glucose measurements, this approach may incorrectly attribute improvement to an otherwise unaltered state. The authors acknowledge that only 4.7% of the contributing studies were randomised controlled trials, and the level of evidence was generally poor (1.6% (10/621) studies assessed as contributing class 1 evidence as per CEBM criteria).

Yip and colleagues performed a large meta-analysis including all studies that reported on diabetes outcomes following either gastric bypass or sleeve gastrectomy.[30] Inclusion criteria used to identify suitable studies were the recruitment of patients aged 18 years or over, the presence of type 2 diabetes prior to bariatric surgery, participants undergoing either gastric bypass or sleeve gastrectomy, and the reporting of glycaemic outcomes with specified criteria at comparable time points of assessment. On this basis, 2655 studies were assessed, of which 33 were considered appropriate for inclusion. The majority of these (30, 18 prospective and 12 retrospective) were not randomised, and 31/33 studies compared either gastric bypass or sleeve gastrectomy against a lifestyle/medical therapy "control" group. 2 of the randomised controlled studies compared gastric bypass against sleeve gastrectomy. Reflective of the available literature reporting on diabetes outcomes following bariatric surgery, only 8/35 studies of outcomes following gastric bypass and 1/16 studies of outcomes following sleeve gastrectomy had a duration of follow up of >12 months. Reported definitions of glycaemic outcome required an HbA1c level below a specified threshold in the absence of glucose lowering therapy.

Using this definition, diabetes remission was achieved by 67% and 56% in those who had undergone gastric bypass and sleeve gastrectomy respectively at 3 months, 76% and 68% at

12 months, and 81% and 80% at 36 months. The authors noted that the differing definition of diabetes remission used had a significant effect on reported outcomes; in those participants who had undergone sleeve gastrectomy, collective studies that defined diabetes remission as an HbA1c <6.0% (42 mmol/mol), <6.5% (47 mmol/mol) or <7.0% (53 mmol/mol) reported diabetes remission in 44.0%, 67.8% and 75.8% of participants respectively.

Conclusion

Early improvements in glucose homeostasis were noted soon after the first bariatric procedures were performed, and a huge volume of evidence validating this phenomenon has since been published. Whilst the study quality and design has varied considerably, the overall assessment of this literature strongly supports bariatric surgery as valid treatment option for obese persons with type 2 diabetes. Indeed, in well designed randomised controlled trials, bariatric surgery is far superior to conventional lifestyle and medical therapy in terms of achieving improvements in glycaemic status alone. Studies presented in this chapter that included a lifestyle/medical arm illustrate the difficulty in achieving improvements in diabetes control that could constitute remission even in a research setting; when stringent criteria for diabetes remission were applied, on average 10% or less of participants in these arms achieved diabetes remission. These findings are clearly of high importance when considering the relative benefit of bariatric surgery in comparison to other treatment options for the management of type 2 diabetes in obese persons.

The marked study heterogeneity with respect to criteria and severity of type 2 diabetes at recruitment, BMI at baseline, specific bariatric procedure performed (even amongst studies purportedly studying the same bariatric modality), definitions of glycaemic outcomes utilised, and concurrent use of medical/lifestyle therapies, means that an absolute stratification of each bariatric procedure to the relative impact on glycaemic control is not possible. Nonetheless, the suggestion of a trend of increasing benefit on glycaemic control with gastric banding (diabetes remission/control at greater than 12 months follow up, seen in 17-73% of included studies), sleeve gastrectomy (11-85%), gastric bypass (24-93%), and biliopancreatic diversion (30-100%) is in keeping with the increasing weight loss seen respectively with each of these procedures in the published literature. In many respects, the interest lies in the analysis of studies reporting on sleeve gastrectomy and gastric bypass as these two procedures are perhaps more comparable than other bariatric procedures. With one exception (Vidal et al, where 85% diabetes remission rates were seen in both arms), all other studies that included both gastric bypass and sleeve gastrectomy, showed improved rates of diabetes remission in those who had undergone gastric bypass. Indeed, this relationship was preserved when one considers outcomes at each follow up interval with improved diabetes remission rates following gastric bypass at 12 months (42-93% versus 23-85% in those undergoing gastric bypass and sleeve gastrectomy respectively), 24 months (33 versus 11%, one study reported [12]) and greater than 24 months (38 versus 24%, one study reported [23]). Whether this apparent benefit on glycaemic outcome of gastric bypass against sleeve gastrectomy translates into clinically meaningful improvements remains to be clarified, as significant reductions in body weight alone are seen following either procedure.

Understandably, many physicians treating patients with type 2 diabetes have historically been reluctant to refer these patients for bariatric surgery, given a paucity of published data on longer term outcomes. This is especially true of younger patients, where the expected long lifespan following surgery clearly increases the risk that any longer term consequences of surgery may negatively affect outcomes. The studies presented above go some way to providing reassurance in this respect, and whilst well designed studies assessing the longer term effect of bariatric surgery on glycaemic complications such as nephropathy, retinopathy, cardiovascular disease are needed, longer term effects on glycaemic status alone are clearly impressive when compared with other currently available therapies. Many authors feel that the more pertinent contemporary question is not if bariatric surgery should at the forefront of therapeutic strategies for obese persons with type 2 diabetes, but at how early it should be performed. Inclusion criteria for many publically funded bariatric surgery programmes internationally select on the presence of more rather than fewer obesity or diabetes related complications; increasing evidence as to the long term efficacy and safety of bariatric procedures would surely therefore require that this approach is reassessed.

In summary, whilst the degree of improvement varies across the published literature, in part because of consistent inconsistencies in the definitions used, the evidence thus far supports a significant and clinically important durable effect of bariatric surgery on glycaemic status. Control groups included in these studies highlight the difficulty in achieving these results without bariatric surgery, even in the context of intensive research based lifestyle and medical interventions. Further research is required to assess the longterm impact on other diabetes related outcomes, but, as per recent statements from the International diabetes federation (IDF), bariatric surgery should now be considered early in the management of obese persons with type 2 diabetes. [1]

References

[1] Zimmet P, Alberti KGMM, Rubino F, Dixon JB. IDF's view of bariatric surgery in type 2 diabetes. *Lancet.* 2011;378(9786):108–10.

[2] Dixon JB, Roux CW, Rubino F, Zimmet P. Bariatric surgery for type 2 diabetes. *Lancet.* 2012;379(9833):2300–2311.

[3] Ihnat M, Thorpe JE, et al. Hypothesis: the "metabolic memory", the new challenge of diabetes. *Diabet Med.* 2007;24(6):582–6.

[4] Holman RR, Paul SK, Bethel MA, Matthews DR, Neil HAW. 10-Year Follow-Up of Intensive Glucose Control in Type 2 Diabetes. *N Engl J Med.* 2008;359(15):1577–89.

[5] Buse JB, Caprio S, Cefalu WT et al. How do we define cure of diabetes? *Diabetes care.* 2009;32(11):2133-2135.

[6] Hofsø D, Nordstrand N, Johnson LK, et al. Obesity-related cardiovascular risk factors after weight loss: a clinical trial comparing gastric bypass surgery and intensive lifestyle intervention. *Eur J Endocrinol.* 2010;163(5):735–45.

[7] Ikramuddin S, Korner J, Lee W-J, et al. Roux-en-Y Gastric Bypass vs Intensive Medical Management for the Control of Type 2 Diabetes, hypertension, and hyperlipidaemia. *JAMA.* 2013;309(21):2240–2249..

[8] Serrot FJ, Dorman RB, Miller CJ, et al. Comparative effectiveness of bariatric surgery and nonsurgical therapy in adults with type 2 diabetes mellitus and body mass index <35 kg/m2. Surgery. 2011;150(4):684–91.

[9] Lee W-J, Chong K, Ser K-H, et al. Gastric Bypass vs Sleeve Gastrectomy for Type 2 Diabetes Mellitus. *Arch Surg*. 2011;146(2):143–148.

[10] Schauer PR, Kashyap SR, Wolski K, et al. Bariatric Surgery versus Intensive Medical Therapy in Obese Patients with Diabetes. *N Engl J Med*. 2012:1–10.

[11] Vidal J, et al. Type 2 Diabetes Mellitus and the Metabolic Syndrome Following Sleeve Gastrectomy in Severely Obese Subjects. *Obes Surg*. 2008;18(9):1077-1082

[12] Kashyap SR, Bhatt DL, Wolski K, et al. Metabolic Effects of Bariatric Surgery. *Diabetes care*. 2013;36:2175–2182.

[13] Scopinaro N, Adami GF, Papadia FS, et al. Effects of biliopanceratic diversion on type 2 diabetes in patients with BMI 25 to 35. *Ann Surg*. 2011;253(4):699–703.

[14] Leslie DP, et al. Efficacy of the Roux-en-Y Gastric Bypass Compared to Medically Managed Controls in Meeting the American Diabetes Association Composite End Point Goals for Management of Type 2 Diabetes Mellitus. *Obes Surg*. 2012;22(3):367-374

[15] Adams TD, Davidson LE, Litwin SE, et al. Health Benefits of Gastric Bypass Surgery After 6 Years. *JAMA*. 2012;308(11).

[16] Dixon JB, O'Brien PE, Playfair J, et al. Adjustable gastric banding and conventional therapy for type 2 diabetes: a randomized controlled trial. *JAMA*. 2008;299(3):316–323.

[17] Sjöström L, Lindroos A, Peltonen M. Lifestyle, diabetes, and cardiovascular risk factors 10 years after bariatric surgery. *N Engl J Med*. 2004;351(26):2683–2693.

[18] Mingrone G, Panunzi S, Gaetano A De, et al. Bariatric Surgery versus Conventional Medical Therapy for Type 2 Diabetes. *N Engl J Med*. 2012:1–9.

[19] Iaconelli A, Panunzi S, De Gaetano A, et al. Effects of bilio-pancreatic diversion on diabetic complications: a 10-year follow-up. *Diabetes Care*. 2011;34(3):561–7..

[20] Pontiroli A, Folli F, Paganelli M, et al. Laparoscopic Gastric Banding Prevents Type 2 Diabetes and Arterial Hypertension and Induces Their Remission in Morbid Obesity. *Diabetes Care*. 2005;28(11):2703–2709.

[21] Pinheiro JS, et al. Long-long limb Roux-en-Y gastric bypass is more efficacious in treatment of type 2 diabetes and lipid disorders in super-obese patients. *Surg Obes Relat Dis*. 2008, 4(4), 521-525

[22] Pournaras DJ, Osborne A, Hawkins SC, Royce P. Remission of Type 2 Diabetes After Gastric Bypass and Banding. *Ann Surg*. 2010;252(6):1–6.

[23] Schauer PR, Bhatt DL, Kirwan JP, et al. Bariatric Surgery versus Intensive Medical Therapy for Diabetes - 3-Year Outcomes. *N Engl J Med*. 2014:1–12.

[24] Li J-F, Lai D-D, Ni B, et al. Comparison of laparoscopic Roux-en-Y gastric bypass with laparoscopic sleeve gastrectomy for morbid obesity or type 2 diabetes mellitus : a meta-analysis of randomized controlled trials. *J Can Chir*. 2013;56(6):158–164.

[25] Maggard-gibbons M, Maglione M, Livhits M, Ewing B, Maher AR. Bariatric Surgery for Weight Loss and Glycemic Control in Nonmorbidly Obese Adults with Diabetes. *JAMA*. 2013;309(21):2250–2261.

[26] Gloy VL, Briel M, Bhatt DL, et al. Bariatric surgery versus non-surgical treatment for obesity : a systematic review and meta-analysis of. *BMJ* 2013;347(October):1–16.

[27] Parikh M, Issa R, Vieira D, et al. Role of bariatric surgery as treatment for type 2 diabetes in patients who do not meet current NIH criteria: a systematic review and meta-analysis. *J Am Coll Surg*. 2013;217(3):527–32.
[28] Buchwald H, Estok R, Fahrbach K, Banel D, et al. Weight and Type 2 Diabetes after Bariatric Surgery : Systematic Review and Meta-analysis. *AJM*. 2009;122(3):248–256.
[29] Buchwald H, Avidor Y, Braunwald E, et al. Bariatric Surgery: A Systematic Review and Meta-analysis. *JAMA*. 2004;292(14):1724–1737.
[30] Yip S, Plank L, Murphy R. Gastric bypass and sleeve gastrectomy for type 2 diabetes: a systematic review and meta-analysis of outcomes. *Obes Surg* 2013:23(12), 1994-2003
[31] Sjostrom L. Review of the key results from the Swedish Obese Subjects (SOS) trial – a prospective controlled intervention study of bariatric surgery. *J Intern Med* 2013; 273: 219–234.

In: Bariatric Surgery
Editor: Mandy Chambers

ISBN: 978-1-63463-697-1

Chapter 5

Adjustable Gastric Banding Surgery: Impact on Inflammation and Iron Metabolism

Cristina Catarino*[1,2], *Susana Coimbra*[2,3], *Luís Belo*[1,2], *Luís Monteiro*[4], *Elísio Costa*[1,2] and *Alice Santos-Silva*[1,2]

[1]Laboratório de Bioquímica, Departamento de Ciências Biológicas, Faculdade de Farmácia, Universidade do Porto (FFUP), Porto, Portugal
[2]Instituto de Biologia Molecular e Celular, IBMC, Universidade do Porto, Porto, Portugal
[3]CESPU, Instituto de Investigação e Formação Avançada em Ciências e Tecnologias da Saúde, GRD-Paredes, Portugal
[4]Hospital da Prelada-Dr. Domingos Braga da Cruz, Porto, Portugal

Abstract

Obesity is increasing all over the world both in developed and underdeveloped countries and is known to be associated with inflammatory changes, insulin resistance and with a hyperlipidemic state. The adipocyte is an important source of adipokines, such as adiponectin, leptin, interleukin (IL)-6 and tumor necrosis factor alpha, and their levels are significantly altered in the plasma of obese patients. Some of these adipokines are known to be associated with dyslipidemia, insulin resistance, vascular dysfunction, and inflammation, and seem to contribute to the development of cardiovascular disease (CVD). Moreover, some inflammatory markers, such as C-reactive protein (CRP), show an independent positive association with body mass index (BMI), and with increased CVD risk.

Cardiovascular morbidity and mortality is associated with the classic risk factors, dyslipidemia, hypertension and impaired glucose metabolism. More recently, inflammatory mechanisms have been accepted as important players in the development of atherosclerotic vascular disease. Obesity, an inflammatory condition, is also an important CVD risk factor.

Recently, it was found that the adipose tissue also expresses hepcidin, and, therefore, may have a direct involvement in iron metabolism. Indeed, obesity is also known to be associated with iron deficiency. The synthesis of hepcidin, an acute phase protein that regulates iron availability, is enhanced in obesity, through IL-6 and leptin secretion by adipose tissue, and may lead to iron deficiency.

Gastric band surgery is a safe surgical procedure for the treatment of morbid obesity, almost without mortality in the perioperative period and a low long-term mortality rate from unrelated causes. Using laparoscopic surgery a gradual, continuous and well-programmed weight loss, is achieved, as well as, a post-operative increasing quality of life and the co-morbidities associated with obesity are also reduced in 75% of patients.

In this book chapter, we will focus on the relationship between obesity, adipose tissue, inflammation and iron metabolism, and we will discuss the impact of gastric banding in the cross-talk between these important factors in obesity.

Introduction

According to the World Health Organization (WHO), obesity affects 35% of the population, [1] and its prevalence is rapidly increasing worldwide, both in developed and underdeveloped countries. Its development has been associated with genetic and environmental factors. Considering that eating habits, with high caloric diets, sedentary lifestyle and reduced levels of physical activity contribute significantly for weight gain, and that the genetics of populations did not change significantly in the last years, the environmental component appears to be very important for the actual obesity prevalence.

Body mass index (BMI) is a simple index, commonly used to classify underweight, overweight and obesity in adults. According to a recent study, [2] individuals with a BMI of 22.5–25.0 kg/m^2 had a normal survival, while individuals with moderate (BMI of 30.0-35.0 kg/m^2) and extreme obesity (BMI of 40.0-50.0 kg/m^2) presented a reduction in life expectancy of 3 and 10 years, respectively. There are several measurements for abdominal adiposity, namely, waist circumference (WC), [3] waist:hip ratio [4]and waist:height ratio. [5] The BMI might be misleading when measuring abdominal adiposity as individuals with a normal BMI may present a large WC. The evaluation of abdominal adiposity is important due to its association with several metabolic dysfunctions, such as, glucose intolerance, reduced insulin sensitivity and adverse lipid profiles.

Actually, obesity, especially abdominal obesity, is considered a strong risk factor for insulin resistance and, as a consequence, for type 2 diabetes *mellitus* (T2DM), [6] as well as, for cardiovascular disease (CVD) events. [7] Obesity has been associated also with inflammatory changes and an hyperlipidemic state, besides insulin resistance, and with an increased risk of CVD events. A hallmark of aging in humans is an increase of adipose mass, especially visceral adipose mass, which is an independent risk factor for chronic heart failure in older people. [8] Moreover, obesity increases the risk of ischemic heart disease, stroke, hypertension, obstructive sleep apnea, degenerative joint conditions, and multiple cancers. [9]

Cardiovascular morbidity and mortality is associated with the classic risk factors, namely dyslipidemia, hypertension and impaired glucose metabolism. However, more recently, inflammatory mechanisms were recognized as playing a vital role in initiation, maintenance and progression of atherosclerotic vascular disease. Atherosclerosis is an inflammatory disease with the participation of leukocytes and several cytokines.

Adipose tissue is an active endocrine organ that secretes several cytokines, known as adipokines. Most of these adipokines are known to interfere with insulin resistance, glucose and lipid metabolism and with the inflammatory process, [10] favoring CVD. Moreover, obesity usually presents a low-grade chronic inflammation, with increased levels of several pro-inflammatory cytokines and acute phase reactants, such as tumour necrosis factor (TNF)-α, interleukin (IL)-1, IL-6 and C-reactive protein (CRP), that are positively correlated with BMI. [11, 12] Therefore, the prevention of obesity assumes a particular importance in human health, quality of life and longevity.

Obesity and Adipokines

Adipokines contribute to appetite regulation and energy expenditure and play an important role in insulin sensitivity, oxidative capacity and lipid uptake. However, in obesity, the amount and characteristics of the adipose tissue is altered, promoting changes in adipokine profile. With obesity, the adipocytes become hypertrophic, inducing hypoxia and an inflammatory response. Moreover, the enhancement of adipose tissue leads to increased macrophage infiltration. Macrophages of the adipose tissue are likely to be an important source of pro-inflammatory cytokines, such as TNF-α and IL-6. [13, 14] It is known that expansion of the adipose tissue during weight gain leads to a recruitment of macrophages into the adipose tissue. [15] Apparently, macrophage infiltration of the white adipose tissue increases with BMI and with adipocyte hypertrophy. [16, 17] The increase in fat mass is associated with alterations in the adipokine profile, favoring hypertension, insulin resistance, dyslipidemia, inflammation and atherogenesis (Figure 1). Herein we will review some of the adipokines, especially their role in inflammation, iron metabolism and CVD risk.

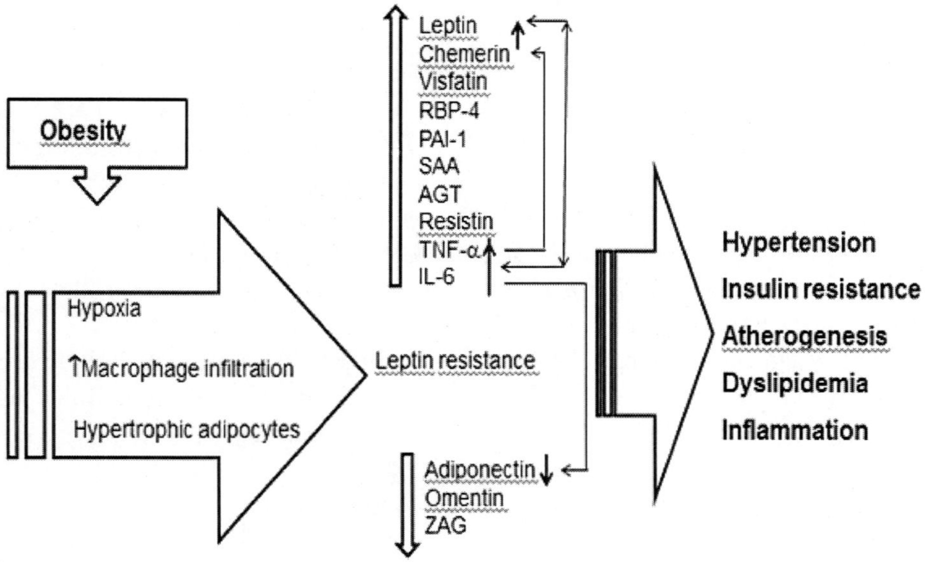

Figure 1. Obesity, adipokine profile and related comorbidities. (AGT, angiotensinogen; IL, interleukin; PAI-1, plasminogen activator inhibitor-1; RBP-4, retinol biding protein-4; SAA, serum amyloid A; TNF-α, tumor necrosis factor-α; ZAG, zinc-α2-glycoprotein).

Leptin controls adipose tissue growth via its central nervous system. Leptin controls food intake, by reducing appetite, body weight and fat stores; their blood levels increase with body fat mass. High levels of leptin enhance T-helper (Th)1 immune responses, suppress Th2 immune responses and increase macrophage activity, with production of different cytokines, namely, TNF-α and IL-6, [18] contributing to the low grade inflammatory state, commonly associated with obesity. It also interferes with antioxidant capacity, increasing reactive oxygen-species (ROS) production and inducible nitric oxide-synthase (iNOS) synthesis. Reduction in leptin activity leads to severe insulin resistance and vascular dysfunction. [18, 19] Leptin levels are known to be enhanced in obesity, [20] however, it seems that a resistance to leptin develops, explaining its reduced activity in obesity. [20] Leptin resistance can be explained by several mechanisms, including defects in leptin transport across the blood–brain barrier, impaired neuronal leptin signaling in target neurons or altered signaling in downstream target cells and neurocircuits. [21]

Chemerin is also an adipose tissue cytokine that has been associated with inflammation, adipogenesis, and with glucose and lipid metabolisms. [22, 23] It has a crucial role in adipocyte differentiation and development, and it may act as a modulator of different metabolic pathways in the mature adipocyte. [23, 24] Chemerin appears to act as modulator of the expression of adipocyte genes involved in glucose and lipid homeostasis. [23] Moreover, chemerin has been associated with several metabolic syndrome markers, namely, increased BMI, triglycerides, blood pressure and insulin resistance. [25] Furthermore, it was recently observed that insulin resistance seems to be a predictor of chemerin levels, independently of BMI. [26]

Visfatin is mainly produced by visceral white adipose tissue. Plasma visfatin is increased in subjects with obesity, T2DM, metabolic syndrome and CVD. [27] Circulating visfatin was positively associated with insulin resistance and hyperglycemia. On the other hand, visfatin appears atherogenic because it contributes to leukocyte adhesion [28] and to atherogenic plaque instability, [29] and may have a direct role in vascular dysfunction and inflammation through iNOS upregulation. [30]

Retinol-binding protein-4 (RBP-4), belongs to the lipocalin family, contributes to insulin resistance and it has been reported that it is increased in human obesity, T2DM and in subclinical atherosclerosis. [31] A positive relationship was found with insulin-resistance severity in obesity, with glucose-intolerance and type 2 diabetes, as well as, with a strong family background for T2DM in non-obese subjects. [32, 33] Lipocalin-2, another lipocalin family member, is an adipokine that has a potential role in insulin resistance and atherosclerosis. [31] The gene and protein expressions of lipocalin-2 in visceral adipose tissue is associated positively with inflammation. [34]

Plasminogen activator inhibitor (PAI)-1 is responsible for decreased fibrinolytic capacity and is, therefore, a cardiovascular risk factor. Ma et al. [35] showed that PAI-1 is increased in obesity and may have a direct role in obesity and in insulin resistance.

Serum amyloid A (SAA), an adipokine released primarily by adipocytes, is significantly increased in obesity and is associated with systemic inflammation and atherosclerosis. [36, 37]

Angiotensinogen undergoes two sequential cleavages by renin and angiotensin converting enzyme to produce angiotensin I and angiotensin II, which plays a major role in blood pressure regulation through salt reabsorption in renal tubules and vasoconstriction.

Adipose-derived angiotensinogen is substantially increased in obese humans, [38] explaining the relationship between systemic hypertension and obesity.

Apelin is an adipokine with a favourable effect on metabolism, due to its positive effect on blood pressure and cardiac contractility. [39] Its secretion appears to be linked to insulin secretion; actually, peripheral apelin injection in obese insulin-resistant mice improved insulin sensitivity and glucose uptake in skeletal muscle. [40] However, increased plasma concentrations of apelin were found in obese hyperinsulinemic and T2DM. [41] Moreover, circulating apelin concentration is not correlated to BMI, [42] suggesting that obesity is not the main determinant to increase plasma apelin. Inflammation and oxidative stress may explain the changes in plasma apelin observed in obesity. [41]

Adipocyte-fatty acid binding protein seems to play a crucial role in diabetes and atherosclerotic disease progress; it is, therefore, proposed as a predictor of the metabolic syndrome [43] and of CVD. [44]

Resistin is expressed by cells of the stromal compartment of the adipose tissue, particularly, by macrophages and by peripheral monocytes that are up-regulated during their differentiation to macrophages. It was named for its ability to induce insulin resistance [45] and some studies support also the association of resistin with obesity. [46] High resistin levels are reported to be associated with atherosclerosis, and it has been shown that resistin increases the expression of several pro-inflammatory cytokines, including TNF-α and IL-6. [47] The correlation between BMI and resistin levels [48] is weak; nonetheless, the proportion of mononuclear leucocytes within adipose tissue correlates well with BMI. [15]

The pro-inflammatory state and the impaired immunity in obesity contribute to increase the levels of several cytokines, such as TNF-α and IL-6. TNF-α is known as a key player in inflammatory cell activation and recruitment. [49] It has been linked to insulin resistance in skeletal muscle and adipose tissue, [50] and it seems to favor atherosclerosis through induction of adhesion molecule expression in endothelial and vascular smooth muscle cells. [51] Moreover, TNF-α induces a strong activation of NF-KB (nuclear factor kappa-light-chain-enhancer of activated B cells), a vital transcription factor that regulates an array of genes associated with inflammation. [52] It was reported that obese individuals, as compared with non-obese, present higher blood levels of TNF-α and soluble TNF-α receptors. The subsets of T cell populations and their function may be reduced in human obesity, and this may be related, at least in part, to the increased TNF-α production. [53]

In the absence of inflammation, the adipose tissue seems to contribute to 15–30% of circulating IL-6. [54] IL-6 impairs insulin stimulation, induces liver production of CRP, and associates with obesity-related hypertriglyceridemia by stimulating hepatic secretion of very low-density lipoproteins. [55, 56] The production of CRP, one of the most sensitive markers of inflammation, results from the interaction of pro-inflammatory cytokines (especially, IL-6, TNF-α and IL-1) with their receptors and inhibitors. Raised concentrations of CRP are thought to be emerging risk factors for CVD. [57] CRP levels are also raised in obesity, and weight loss usually leads to a reduction in CRP. [58]

Obesity associates with increased levels of some adipokines, but also with a decrease in the production of others. Adiponectin has anti-inflammatory activity and a protective role against insulin resistance. Adiponectin is inversely associated with the adhesion molecule expression and the transformation of macrophages into foam cells. It seems to protect against metabolic diseases and also against atherosclerosis. [59, 60] However, the protective role for

CVD is controversial, with several data reporting a positive association of adiponectin with risk for all-cause and cardiovascular mortality. [61-63] Higher adiponectin levels were strongly associated with a lower risk of impaired glucose metabolism and T2DM, suggesting that adiponectin is involved in their pathophysiology, linking obesity to T2DM. [64] The obese patients, especially those with visceral obesity, seem to present decreased plasma concentrations of adiponectin. [65, 66] This, suggests the existence of a feedback inhibition process, working when the total body fat mass increases, and inducing an increase in the secretion of other adipokines or a decrease in the metabolic function of the adipocyte. [67]

Omentin is strongly expressed in stromal vascular cells of adipose tissue, and seems to have a role in modulating insulin action. [68] It appears to have anti-inflammatory ability, reducing endothelial dysfunction and atherosclerosis. [69] Obese or overweight individuals have lower plasma omentin levels when compared with lean subjects [70] and its levels are inversely correlated with BMI, WC and circulating leptin. [70, 71] Omentin is also decreased in patients with coronary artery disease. [72]

Zinc-α2-glycoprotein (ZAG) seems to correlate inversely with markers of obesity such as BMI and WC. [73, 74] Although the factors that down-regulate ZAG are not well understood, obesity-related inflammation could be involved in its regulation. ZAG may act like adiponectin in protecting against the obese state. [75, 76]

Vaspin (visceral adipose tissue-derived serine protease inhibitor) is an adipokine expressed in visceral white adipose tissue. Fat mass expansion has been associated with increased expression of vaspin and its circulating levels. [77, 78] In obese subjects, serum vaspin decreases following a modest weight loss, which is accompanied by improvement in insulin resistance. [79] However, the mechanisms by which vaspin secretion is linked to glucose metabolism and to insulin sensitivity are not entirely understood. Administration of vaspin to obese mice improves glucose tolerance, insulin sensitivity, and reduces food intake. Until now molecular target(s) of vaspin and its mode of action are unknown. [80]

Some adipokines interfere in the regulation of each other's. For instance, TNF-α and IL-6 are involved in the regulation of other adipokines, such as adiponectin; [81] leptin and chemerin production is stimulated by TNF-α. [82]

In summary, in obesity, there is hypoxia, increased macrophage infiltration and adipocytes are hypertrophic and resistant to leptin and insulin action. Although the role of some adipokines is not completely known, the adipokine profile in obesity changes, usually presenting an increase in the levels of leptin, chemerin, visfatin, RBP-4, PAI-1, SAA, angiotensinogen, resistin, TNF-α and IL-6, and a reduction in adiponectin, omentin and ZAG (Figure 1). These changes seem to favor hypertension, insulin resistance, atherogenesis, dyslipidemia and inflammation.

The Impact of Gastric Banding Surgery in Obesity and Related Comorbidities

According to the current guidelines, bariatric surgery is recommended for patients with a BMI > 40 kg/m^2 and for patients with a BMI 35-40 kg/m^2, when presenting serious comorbidities associated with obesity, such as hypertension, diabetes or hypercholesterolemia. [83, 84]

Laparoscopic adjustable gastric banding (LAGB), sleeve gastrectomy and Roux-en-Y gastric bypass are techniques used in bariatric surgery; this surgery has been very successful in morbid obesity as it has been shown to be more effective than lifestyle intervention (physical activity, diet and weight reducing drugs). [85]

Using LAGB surgery a gradual, continuous and well-programmed weight loss, is achieved; moreover, it increases the quality of life of the patients and reduces co-morbidities in over 75% of patients, including the systemic inflammatory response. [86] Laparoscopic surgery, compared with the conventional open method, is mini-invasive and has decreased postoperative pain and length of hospitalization. It is associated with lower rates of complications, lower hospital readmission, and lower mortality. [87, 88]

LAGB is the most common surgery, as it is the easiest surgical technique. It involves the placement of an adjustable gastric band around the upper stomach. The gastric band is connected to an inflatable balloon that can be adjusted by adding or removing saline via a small subcutaneous access port. A loss of 47% excess weight may be maintained for about 15 years, as it shows a substantial long-term weight loss, which is similar to other bariatric procedures. [89] Several studies showed that the laparoscopic gastric band surgery in morbidly obese patients lead to a significant weight loss, [90, 91] even after a short period of one month. [90] Moreover, several authors documented a medium to long-term sustained weight loss with laparoscopic adjustable band gastric. [92-96]

Some authors reported [97] that the other bariatric techniques provide a higher degree of weight loss, however, LAGB seems to be associated with less and fewer severe complications. [98, 99]

Significant improvements in health-related quality of life (HRQOL) have been reported, even in the first year after LAGB. [100] A poor baseline HRQOL, a high efficacy of the banding in controlling eat disorders, and a higher weight loss, are believed to be important factors to improve HRQOL of the patients. [100]

Resolution of obesity-related comorbidities depends on significant and sustained weight loss and on excess weight loss. [101, 102] According to Brancatisano et al., [103] weight loss, after Swedish adjustable gastric band placement, is an effective treatment of T2DM in morbidly obese patients. In this case, an early intervention offers the greatest chance of remission.

The authors suggested that it might even prevent the occurrence of T2DM in patients with impaired glucose tolerance. [103] Indeed, it was reported that the extensive weight loss in formerly obese women, after Swedish adjustable gastric band surgery, was accompanied by an increase in insulin sensitivity, as showed by fasting insulin and the HOMA index; these favorable metabolic changes were also observed in women after a successful weight loss, by diet alone but were less pronounced. [104]

The LAGB induces a substantial sustained positive effect on diabetes in morbidly obese patients, with a significant reduction in glycated hemoglobin (HbA1c) levels and a combined improvement/remission rate of 80%. [105]

Table 1. Main findings reported in studies in obese patients after laparoscopic adjustable gastric banding (LAGB) surgery

Study	Obese Subjects	Follow up after LAGB surgery	Main Findings (*)	
Hanusch-Enserer et al. (2004) [121]	18 patients (15 F / 3 M)	6 months	↓ BMI, WC, DBP, SBP, glucose, C-peptide, TG, leptin, insulin	
		12 months	↓ BMI, WC, DBP, SBP, C-peptide, TG, GPT, γ-GT, leptin, insulin	↑ ghrelin
Coupaye et al. (2005) [144]	36 women	12 months	↓ fat mass, lean body mass, leptin	
Ram et al. (2005) [111]	23 patients (15 F / 8 M)	6 months	↓ BMI, insulin, proinsulin, leptin	
		14 months	↓ BMI, insulin, proinsulin, leptin	
Diker et al. (2006) [145]	23 patients (15 F / 8 M)	6 months	↓ BMI	↑ adiponectin
		14 months	↓ BMI	↑ adiponectin
Gasteyger et al. (2006) [129]	36 women (premenopausal) LAGB + Swedish LAGB	6 months	↓ BMI, fat, fat free mass, DBP, SBP, glucose, TChol, TG	↑ MCV; No alteration: iron and ferritin
		12 months	↓ BMI, fat, fat free mass, DBP, SBP, glucose, TChol, TG	↑ HDLc, MCV; No alteration: iron and ferritin
		18 months	↓ BMI, fat, fat free mass, DBP, SBP, glucose, TChol, TG, Hb	↑ HDLc; No alteration: iron and ferritin
		24 months	↓ BMI, fat, fat free mass, DBP, SBP, glucose, TChol, TG, Hb	↑ HDLc; No alteration: iron and ferritin
Anty et al. (2008) [143]	55 female patients "Roux en Y" gastric bypass + vertical calibrated gastroplasties + LAGB	6 months	↓ BMI, CRP, Orosomucoid	↑ TrSat
Shak et al. (2008) [112]	24 patients (14F / 10M)	6 months	↓ BMI, leptin	No alteration: total ghrelin, acylated ghrelin, insulin
		12 months	↓ BMI, leptin	No alteration: total ghrelin, acylated ghrelin, insulin

Study	Obese Subjects	Follow up after LAGB surgery	Main Findings (*)	
Korner et al. (2009) [114]	15 patients (11 F / 4 M)	2 weeks	↓ leptin, insulin, glucose, HOMA-IR	No alteration: PYY, ghrelin, GLP-1
		12 weeks	↓ leptin	No alteration: PYY, ghrelin, GLP-1
		26 weeks	↓ leptin, insulin, glucose, HOMA-IR	No alteration: PYY, ghrelin, GLP-1
		52 weeks	↓ leptin, insulin, glucose, HOMA-IR	No alteration: PYY, ghrelin, GLP-1
Moschen et al. (2009) [113]	30 patients (24 F / 6 M)	6 months	↓ BMI, glucose, insulin, HOMA-IR, CRP, TNF-α, leptin, PBEF/Nampt/visfatin	↑ adiponectin, resistin
		12 months	↓ BMI, glucose, insulin, HOMA-IR, CRP, TNF-α, leptin, resistin, PBEF/Nampt/visfatin	↑ adiponectin
Ramalho et al. (2009) [126]	32 women	1 month	↓ BMI, CRP, haptoglobin, transferrin, LDLc, TChol	↑ Alfa-1 antitrypsin, ferritin, sTFR, HDLc
		18 months	↓ BMI, glucose, CRP, haptoglobin, ferritin, sTFR	↑ Alfa-1 antitrypsin, transferrin, LDLc, TChol, HDLc
Trakhtenbroit et al. (2009)106	5 women	3 months	↓ insulin, HOMA-IR	No alteration: glucose
		9 months	↓ insulin, HOMA-IR	No alteration: glucose
		24 months		No alteration: glucose, insulin, HOMA-IR
Moschen et al. (2010) [128]	20 severely patients (13 F / 7 M)	6 months	↓ BMI, glucose, insulin, HOMA-IR, TChol, TG, CRP, IL-6	No detectable: TNF-α
Tussing-Humphreys et al. (2010) [109]	20 women LAGB + LSG	6 months	↓ BMI, WC, sTFR, hepcidin, HOMA-IR, CRP, IL-6, EPO	↑Hb, Ht
Benedix et al. (2011) [146]	Obese patients (7 F / 7 M)	6 months	↓ BMI, glucose, insulin	↑ adiponectin; No alteration: insulin, salivary ghrelin
		12 months	↓ BMI, glucose	↑ adiponectin; No alteration: insulin, salivary ghrelin
Marantos et al. (2011)110	20 women LAGB (13) + LSG (7)	12 months	↓ BMI, leptin, resistin, IL-6	↑ adiponectin
Plum et al. (2011) [107]	8 Obese patients (7 F / 1 M)		↓ BMI, insulin, HOMA-IR, c-peptide, leptin, HDLc	

Table 1. (Continued)

Study	Obese Subjects	Follow up after LAGB surgery	Main Findings (*)	
Bradley et al (2012) [108]	10 patients (9 F / 1 M)	22 ± 7 weeks	↓ BMI, glucose, insulin, HOMA-IR, c-peptide, leptin, CRP	↑ adiponectin
Cugno et al. (2012) [127]	25 women	3 months	↓ BMI, CRP, PAI-1, fibrinogen, VWF	
		6 months	↓ BMI, CRP, PAI-1, fibrinogen, VWF	
		12 months	↓ BMI, CRP, PAI-1, fibrinogen, VWF	
Gelisgen et al. (2012) [91]	21 patients (12 F / 9 M)	6 months	↓ BMI, insulin, HOMA-IR;	↑ acylated ghrelin; No alteration: glucose
Hady et al. (2012) [122]	100 patients (66 F / 34 M)	7 days	↓ BMI, insulin,	No alteration: glucose, HOMA-IR, HDLc
		1 month	↓ BMI, ghrelin, insulin,	
		3 months	↓ BMI, ghrelin, insulin, T Chol, LDL, TG	
		6 months	↓ BMI, insulin, T Chol, LDL, TG	
Krieger et al. (2012) [115]	30 patients (20 F / 10 M)	12 months	↓ BMI, leptin	No alteration: ghrelin
Cigdem et al. (2013) [90]	20 patients	1 month	↓ BMI, leptin, orexin-A, insulin resistance	↑ ghrelin
Samaras et al. (2013) [130]	15 patients	2 weeks	↓ BMI, SBP, glucose, insulin, HbA1C, TChol, TG, HDLc, LDLc	
		12 weeks	↓ BMI, SBP, glucose, HbA1C, TG	
Visockiene et al. (2013) [147]	90 patients (61 F / 29 M)	12 months	↓ BMI, fat mass, glucose, HbA1C, TG	↑ HDLc
Santos et al. (2014) [86]	46 patients (40 F / 6 M)	3 months	↓ hsCRP, neutrophil count, TG, transferrin	↑ transferrin saturation; No alteration: iron, ferritin

F, female; M, male.

BMI, body mass index; CRP, C-reactive protein; DBP, diastolic blood pressure; EPO, erythropoietin; GLP-1, Glucagon-like peptide-1; GPT, glutamic pyruvic transaminase; Hb, hemoglobin; HbA1C, glycated hemoglobin; HDLc, high-density lipoprotein cholesterol; HOMA-IR, homeostasis model assessment of insulin resistance; hsCRP, high-sensitivity CRP; Ht, hematocrit; IL, interleukin; LDLc, low-density lipoprotein cholesterol; LSG, laparoscopic sleeve gastrectomy; MCV, mean corpuscular volume; PAI-1, plasminogen activator inhibitor-1; PBEF, pre-B cell enhancing factor; PYY, peptide YY; SBP, systolic blood pressure; sTfR, soluble transferrin receptor; TChol, Total cholesterol; TG, Triglycerides; TNF-α, tumor necrosis factor- α; TrSat, transferrin saturation; VWF, von Willebrand factor; WC, waist circumference; γ-GT; γ-glutamyl transferase.

(*) Findings compared to baseline.

The Impact of LAGB in Adipokines and in the Inflammatory State

As already referred, obesity is characterized by a low grade inflammatory process, involving several inflammatory mediators, produced by the adipose tissue. Conservative weight management techniques, including medication, often fail to achieve substantial and prolonged weight loss and reduction of inflammation in morbid obese individuals, explaining the increase success of bariatric surgery.

In Table 1 are summarized the main findings observed in follow up studies in obese patients, after LAGB surgery.

In general, a marked decrease in weight of morbid obese patients occurs after LAGB surgery. Only a small number of studies focused on the inflammatory profile, adipokines levels or iron status, after LAGB surgery, and most of them provide very limited results. The small sample size is the most frequent limitation of the studies. [106-108] Comparisons between studies are difficult, as they present different periods of follow-up and, sometimes, the follow-up period was insufficient to confirm the long-term effects of bariatric surgery.

Furthermore, some studies cannot be used for comparisons as they included subjects submitted to two different surgery techniques. [109, 110]

Leptin is one of the adipokines that has been studied in obese patients after LAGB surgery. A decrease in leptin levels has been reported, [90, 108, 111-116] as soon as one month after laparascopic gastric band. [90] Ritt et al. [104] reported that women after Swedish adjustable gastric band, showed a significant reduction in leptin, while TNF-α serum levels increased, compared with dietary-treated obese patients.

Few studies exist concerning the changes induced in the novel adipokines, apelin, resistin, RBP-4, vaspin and visfatin, after bariatric surgery. Inconclusive results are described for resistin concentrations; indeed, obese patients, after LAGB surgery, presented higher resistin levels 6 months after surgery; [113] nevertheless, 12 months after surgery resistin levels decreased significantly. [110, 113]

Botella-Carretero et al. [117] reported an increase in visfatin concentration in obese patients after gastric bypass and biliopancreatic diversion surgery. Plasma visfatin levels are also increased in severely obese patients after intestinal bypass. [118]

In summary, more studies are needed to understand the relationship between weight loss imposed by LAGB and the secretion of adipokines, namely of novel adipokines, by the reduced adipose tissue.

Ghrelin, which stimulates appetite and food intake, enhancing fat mass deposition and weight gain, [119] is down-regulated in obesity. [120] Nevertheless contradictory results are reported concerning ghrelin levels after LAGB surgery; while some authors reported an increase in ghrelin [90, 121] and acylated ghrelin levels, [91] others described lower levels [122] or no alteration in ghrelin [114, 115] and acylated ghrelin [112] concentration.

Surgical injury induces a systemic inflammatory metabolic-endocrine response that is proportional to the severity of the surgical stress. The systemic inflammatory response was evaluated at 6 and 12 hours after laparoscopic adjustable gastric banding (were significantly reduced compared with those) and after open stoma-adjustable silicone band application, and it was reported that the inflammatory response was significantly lower for LAGB. [123]

A positive effect on fibrinolytic function, oxidative stress and antioxidant activity, which are associated to obesity, has been achieved with both open and laparoscopic gastric band interventions. Moreover, postoperative BMI, lipid profile, malondialdehyde (MDA), oxidized low-density lipoprotein (oxLDL), leptin and PAI-1 decreased significantly after both surgeries, while paraoxonase activity increased and was negatively correlated with BMI, MDA, oxLDL, leptin and PAI-1. [116] These studies suggest that several positive effects are observed as a result of weight loss after surgery.

After bariatric surgery, the visceral adipose expression of macrophage and T cell markers, by defining the adipose expression of TNF-α and IL-1 receptor antagonist, contribute to the systemic levels of TNF-α and IL-6. A higher inflammatory state of the adipose tissue seems to predict a lower BMI reduction after surgery, notably at early stages after surgery. [124]

Indeed, there is some controversial data about the reduction in the inflammatory profile after gastric band surgery; Keogh et al, reported a 40% reduction in CRP levels one year after Swedish adjustable gastric band surgery. [125]

Other studies showed that as soon as 1 month after LAGB surgery, the obese patients present an improvement in the inflammatory profile, with a reduction in CRP and haptoglobin levels [126] that remain low for 18 months after surgery. Cugno et al. [127] observed a reversion of the low-grade inflammation at 3 months after bariatric surgery. Several other studies reported a reduction in the inflammatory process after weight loss by LAGB surgery, as shown by a decrease in CRP [86, 113, 127] and IL-6 levels. [110, 128]

Besides the improvement in the inflammatory state, insulin resistance and adipokine levels, several studies reported an improvement in the lipid profile [122, 129, 130] and in glucose related markers. [111, 113, 114, 121, 128, 130].

Obesity, Iron Status and the Impact of LAGB on Iron Metabolism

Iron deficiency is the most prevalent worldwide nutritional problem, [131] having significant public health implications. The development of iron deficiency occurs in two stages, starting by depletion of iron stores, followed by depletion of iron containing proteins and enzymes, including hemoglobin, which leads to an overt iron deficiency anemia. Data confirmed an association between obesity and hypoferremia in children, adolescents, adult men and women, and post-menopausal women, in both developed and transitional countries. [132-135]. Considering that iron deficiency seems to diminish cognitive function and exercise performance, the association with obesity may represent a poor prognostic for a healthy physical and psychological condition.

The mechanisms that link iron status and obesity are still poorly clarified. The most accepted hypothesis is that iron deficiency is a consequence of the chronic low-grade inflammation state in obesity.

Hepcidin is a major regulator of iron availability for erythropoiesis. It inhibits iron intestinal absorption and reduces the flux of iron from splenic and hepatic macrophages, [136] as it binds to the cellular iron export channel ferroportin-1, present in enterocytes, hepatocytes and macrophages; ferroportin is needed for iron absoption and iron mobilization. The linkage of hepcidin to ferroportin induces ferroportin internalization and degradation, reducing iron availability. [137] The hepatic transcription of hepcidin is up-regulated by pro-inflammatory cytokines, bone morphogenetic proteins (BMP) and iron overload, and is down-regulated by iron deficiency, ineffective erythropoiesis and hypoxia. [138]

Besides the liver, hepcidin is also expressed in other tissues, namely in the adipose tissue. [139] Indeed, data suggest that adipocytes are capable of producing hepcidin, and this production is probably triggered by inflammatory stimuli. [140, 141] It seems that inflammatory changes in the adipose tissue increase hepcidin expression, which might contribute to the erythropoietic disturbances resulting from changes in iron metabolism that could, ultimately, lead to iron deficiency. [141] However, there are still controversies concerning the contribute of adipocytes to the circulating levels of hepcidin, its importance in obesity and its linkage to erythropoietic disturbances. In healthy individuals, the hepatic hepcidin expression is higher than the adipocyte hepcidin expression; however, in obesity the adipose tissue mass increases and is higher than liver mass; [133] thus, in obesity, the hepcidin secreted by the adipose tissue, may be relevant for iron status and erythropoiesis. Hemojuvelin, which enhances hepcidin expression in the liver, is also expressed in adipocytes and highly increased in adipose tissue from obese. [142] Actually, blood concentrations of soluble hemojuvelin were significantly increased in obese patients, as compared to controls, suggesting that the adipose tissue may have a role in iron homeostasis in obesity and in erythropoiesis. More studies that contribute to clarify the interplay between protein expression-iron status-erythropoiesis are required.

There are few studies concerning the effects of LAGB surgery on iron metabolism. According to Anty et al. [143] bariatric surgery improved iron status in obese patients, as it corrected iron depletion, alongside with the reduction in adipose mass, and inflammation in the patients; Anty et al. [143] also observed a reversion of iron depletion in obese patients 6 months after bariatric surgery; apparently, bariatric surgery improved iron status by reducing chronic inflammation. Actuall~~a~~y, they found a significant negative correlation between CRP levels and transferrin saturation; nevertheless, considering that the bariatric surgery included different techniques, namely vertical calibrated gastroplasties, LAGB and "Roux en Y" gastric bypass, it was difficult to analyze the relationship between iron status and the type of bariatric surgery.

Another study, by performing a follow-up of 3 months after LAGB surgery, reported also an increased in iron availability, as shown by an increase transferrin saturation in obese patients. [86]

In opposition to these findings, a follow up study reported that no alterations were observed in iron and ferritin levels 24 months after LAGB. [129]

Conclusion

LAGB associates with a successful decrease in body weight, an improvement in inflammatory markers, insulin resistance and lipid profile. Regarding adipokines, LAGB induces a decrease in leptin and an increase in adiponectin levels; however, there is a lack in data studying the effect of LAGB in novel adipokines. Concerning ~~to~~ iron bioavailability, further studies are needed to understand the role of the adipose tissue in iron metabolism, in obesity, and the influence of weight loss, imposed by LAGB.

References

[1] WHO. Obesity: Preventing and managing the global epidemic. Report of a WHO Consultation on Obesity; Geneve: WHO; 2000

[2] Whitlock G, Lewington S, Sherliker P, et al. Body-mass index and cause-specific mortality in 900 000 adults: collaborative analyses of 57 prospective studies. *Lancet.* 2009;373(9669):1083-96.

[3] Wei M, Gaskill SP, Haffner SM, Stern MP. Waist circumference as the best predictor of noninsulin dependent diabetes mellitus (NIDDM) compared to body mass index, waist/hip ratio and other anthropometric measurements in Mexican Americans--a 7-year prospective study. *Obes Res.* 1997;5(1):16-23.

[4] Welborn TA, Dhaliwal SS. Preferred clinical measures of central obesity for predicting mortality. *Eur J Clin Nutr.* 2007;61(12):1373-9.

[5] Ashwell M, Hsieh SD. Six reasons why the waist-to-height ratio is a rapid and effective global indicator for health risks of obesity and how its use could simplify the international public health message on obesity. *Int J Food Sci Nutr.* 2005;56(5):303-7.

[6] Koh-Banerjee P, Wang Y, Hu FB, Spiegelman D, Willett WC, Rimm EB. Changes in body weight and body fat distribution as risk factors for clinical diabetes in US men. *Am J Epidemiol.* 2004;159(12):1150-9.

[7] Walker SP, Rimm EB, Ascherio A, Kawachi I, Stampfer MJ, Willett WC. Body size and fat distribution as predictors of stroke among US men. *Am J Epidemiol.* 1996;144(12):1143-50.

[8] Nicklas BJ, Cesari M, Penninx BW, et al. Abdominal obesity is an independent risk factor for chronic heart failure in older people. *J Am Geriatr Soc.* 2006;54(3):413-20.

[9] Haslam DW, James WP. Obesity. *Lancet.* 2005;366(9492):1197-209.

[10] Rondinone CM. Adipocyte-derived hormones, cytokines, and mediators. *Endocrine.* 2006;29(1):81-90.

[11] Wellen KE, Hotamisligil GS. Obesity-induced inflammatory changes in adipose tissue. *J Clin Invest.* 2003;112(12):1785-8.

[12] Panagiotakos DB, Pitsavos C, Yannakoulia M, Chrysohoou C, Stefanadis C. The implication of obesity and central fat on markers of chronic inflammation: The ATTICA study. *Atherosclerosis.* 2005;183(2):308-15.

[13] Fain JN, Madan AK, Hiler ML, Cheema P, Bahouth SW. Comparison of the release of adipokines by adipose tissue, adipose tissue matrix, and adipocytes from visceral and subcutaneous abdominal adipose tissues of obese humans. *Endocrinology.* 2004;145(5):2273-82.

[14] Bruun JM, Lihn AS, Madan AK, et al. Higher production of IL-8 in visceral vs. subcutaneous adipose tissue. Implication of nonadipose cells in adipose tissue. *Am J Physiol Endocrinol Metab.* 2004;286(1):E8-13.

[15] Curat CA, Wegner V, Sengenes C, et al. Macrophages in human visceral adipose tissue: increased accumulation in obesity and a source of resistin and visfatin. *Diabetologia*. 2006;49(4):744-7.

[16] Curat CA, Miranville A, Sengenes C, et al. From blood monocytes to adipose tissue-resident macrophages: induction of diapedesis by human mature adipocytes. *Diabetes*. 2004;53(5):1285-92.

[17] Weisberg SP, McCann D, Desai M, Rosenbaum M, Leibel RL, Ferrante AW, Jr. Obesity is associated with macrophage accumulation in adipose tissue. *J Clin Invest*. 2003;112(12):1796-808.

[18] Santos-Alvarez J, Goberna R, Sanchez-Margalet V. Human leptin stimulates proliferation and activation of human circulating monocytes. *Cell Immunol*. 1999;194(1):6-11.

[19] Zhang Y, Proenca R, Maffei M, Barone M, Leopold L, Friedman JM. Positional cloning of the mouse obese gene and its human homologue. *Nature*. 1994;372(6505):425-32.

[20] Enriori PJ, Evans AE, Sinnayah P, Cowley MA. Leptin resistance and obesity. *Obesity (Silver Spring)*. 2006;14 Suppl 5:254S-8S.

[21] Coppari R, Bjorbaek C. Leptin revisited: its mechanism of action and potential for treating diabetes. *Nat Rev Drug Discov*. 2012;11(9):692-708.

[22] Bozaoglu K, Bolton K, McMillan J, et al. Chemerin is a novel adipokine associated with obesity and metabolic syndrome. *Endocrinology*. 2007;148(10):4687-94.

[23] Goralski KB, McCarthy TC, Hanniman EA, et al. Chemerin, a novel adipokine that regulates adipogenesis and adipocyte metabolism. *J Biol Chem*. 2007;282(38):28175-88.

[24] Roh SG, Song SH, Choi KC, et al. Chemerin--a new adipokine that modulates adipogenesis via its own receptor. *Biochem Biophys Res Commun*. 2007;362(4):1013-8.

[25] Stejskal D, Karpisek M, Hanulova Z, Svestak M. Chemerin is an independent marker of the metabolic syndrome in a Caucasian population--a pilot study. *Biomed Pap Med Fac Univ Palacky Olomouc Czech Repub*. 2008;152(2):217-21.

[26] Chakaroun R, Raschpichler M, Kloting N, et al. Effects of weight loss and exercise on chemerin serum concentrations and adipose tissue expression in human obesity. *Metabolism*. 2012;61(5):706-14.

[27] Chang YH, Chang DM, Lin KC, Shin SJ, Lee YJ. Visfatin in overweight/obesity, type 2 diabetes mellitus, insulin resistance, metabolic syndrome and cardiovascular diseases: a meta-analysis and systemic review. *Diabetes Metab Res Rev*. 2011;27(6):515-27.

[28] Kim SR, Bae YH, Bae SK, et al. Visfatin enhances ICAM-1 and VCAM-1 expression through ROS-dependent NF-kappaB activation in endothelial cells. *Biochim Biophys Acta*. 2008;1783(5):886-95.

[29] Dahl TB, Yndestad A, Skjelland M, et al. Increased expression of visfatin in macrophages of human unstable carotid and coronary atherosclerosis: possible role in inflammation and plaque destabilization. *Circulation*. 2007;115(8):972-80.

[30] Romacho T, Azcutia V, Vazquez-Bella M, et al. Extracellular PBEF/NAMPT/visfatin activates pro-inflammatory signalling in human vascular smooth muscle cells through nicotinamide phosphoribosyltransferase activity. *Diabetologia*. 2009;52(11):2455-63.

[31] Xiao Y, Xu A, Hui X, et al. Circulating lipocalin-2 and retinol-binding protein 4 are associated with intima-media thickness and subclinical atherosclerosis in patients with type 2 diabetes. *PLoS One*. 2013;8(6):e66607.
[32] Graham TE, Yang Q, Bluher M, et al. Retinol-binding protein 4 and insulin resistance in lean, obese, and diabetic subjects. *N Engl J Med*. 2006;354(24):2552-63.
[33] Hammarstedt A, Graham TE, Kahn BB. Adipose tissue dysregulation and reduced insulin sensitivity in non-obese individuals with enlarged abdominal adipose cells. *Diabetol Metab Syndr*. 2012;4(1):42.
[34] Catalan V, Gomez-Ambrosi J, Rodriguez A, et al. Increased adipose tissue expression of lipocalin-2 in obesity is related to inflammation and matrix metalloproteinase-2 and metalloproteinase-9 activities in humans. *J Mol Med (Berl)*. 2009;87(8):803-13.
[35] Ma LJ, Mao SL, Taylor KL, et al. Prevention of obesity and insulin resistance in mice lacking plasminogen activator inhibitor 1. *Diabetes*. 2004;53(2):336-46.
[36] Zhao Y, He X, Shi X, et al. Association between serum amyloid A and obesity: a meta-analysis and systematic review. *Inflamm Res*. 2010;59(5):323-34.
[37] Johnson BD, Kip KE, Marroquin OC, et al. Serum amyloid A as a predictor of coronary artery disease and cardiovascular outcome in women: the National Heart, Lung, and Blood Institute-Sponsored Women's Ischemia Syndrome Evaluation (WISE). *Circulation*. 2004;109(6):726-32.
[38] Yasue S, Masuzaki H, Okada S, et al. Adipose tissue-specific regulation of angiotensinogen in obese humans and mice: impact of nutritional status and adipocyte hypertrophy. *Am J Hypertens*. 2010;23(4):425-31.
[39] Kleinz MJ, Davenport AP. Emerging roles of apelin in biology and medicine. *Pharmacol Ther*. 2005;107(2):198-211.
[40] Yue P, Jin H, Aillaud M, et al. Apelin is necessary for the maintenance of insulin sensitivity. *Am J Physiol Endocrinol Metab*. 2010;298(1):E59-67.
[41] Yu S, Zhang Y, Li MZ, et al. Chemerin and apelin are positively correlated with inflammation in obese type 2 diabetic patients. *Chin Med J (Engl)*. 2012;125(19):3440-4.
[42] Leal VO, Lobo JC, Stockler-Pinto MB, et al. Apelin: a peptide involved in cardiovascular risk in hemodialysis patients? *Ren Fail*. 2012;34(5):577-81.
[43] Xu A, Tso AW, Cheung BM, et al. Circulating adipocyte-fatty acid binding protein levels predict the development of the metabolic syndrome: a 5-year prospective study. *Circulation*. 2007;115(12):1537-43.
[44] Chow WS, Tso AW, Xu A, et al. Elevated circulating adipocyte-fatty acid binding protein levels predict incident cardiovascular events in a community-based cohort: a 12-year prospective study. *J Am Heart Assoc*. 2013;2(1):e004176.
[45] Chen BH, Song Y, Ding EL, et al. Circulating levels of resistin and risk of type 2 diabetes in men and women: results from two prospective cohorts. *Diabetes Care*. 2009;32(2):329-34.
[46] Owecki M, Miczke A, Nikisch E, Pupek-Musialik D, Sowinski J. Serum resistin concentrations are higher in human obesity but independent from insulin resistance. *Exp Clin Endocrinol Diabetes*. 2011;119(2):117-21.
[47] Bokarewa M, Nagaev I, Dahlberg L, Smith U, Tarkowski A. Resistin, an adipokine with potent proinflammatory properties. *J Immunol*. 2005;174(9):5789-95.

[48] Kaser S, Kaser A, Sandhofer A, Ebenbichler CF, Tilg H, Patsch JR. Resistin messenger-RNA expression is increased by proinflammatory cytokines in vitro. *Biochem Biophys Res Commun*. 2003;309(2):286-90.

[49] Clark IA. How TNF was recognized as a key mechanism of disease. *Cytokine Growth Factor Rev*. 2007;18(3-4):335-43.

[50] Lorenzo M, Fernandez-Veledo S, Vila-Bedmar R, Garcia-Guerra L, De Alvaro C, Nieto-Vazquez I. Insulin resistance induced by tumor necrosis factor-alpha in myocytes and brown adipocytes. *J Anim Sci*. 2008;86(14 Suppl):E94-104.

[51] Choy JC, Granville DJ, Hunt DW, McManus BM. Endothelial cell apoptosis: biochemical characteristics and potential implications for atherosclerosis. *J Mol Cell Cardiol*. 2001;33(9):1673-90.

[52] Antunes F, Han D. Redox regulation of NF-kappaB: from basic to clinical research. *Antioxid Redox Signal*. 2009;11(9):2055-6.

[53] Tanaka S, Isoda F, Ishihara Y, Kimura M, Yamakawa T. T lymphopaenia in relation to body mass index and TNF-alpha in human obesity: adequate weight reduction can be corrective. *Clin Endocrinol (Oxf)*. 2001;54(3):347-54.

[54] Mohamed-Ali V, Goodrick S, Rawesh A, et al. Subcutaneous adipose tissue releases interleukin-6, but not tumor necrosis factor-alpha, in vivo. *J Clin Endocrinol Metab*. 1997;82(12):4196-200.

[55] Nieto-Vazquez I, Fernandez-Veledo S, de Alvaro C, Lorenzo M. Dual role of interleukin-6 in regulating insulin sensitivity in murine skeletal muscle. *Diabetes*. 2008;57(12):3211-21.

[56] Sparks JD, Cianci J, Jokinen J, Chen LS, Sparks CE. Interleukin-6 mediates hepatic hypersecretion of apolipoprotein B. *Am J Physiol Gastrointest Liver Physiol*. 2010;299(4):G980-9.

[57] Helfand M, Buckley DI, Freeman M, et al. Emerging risk factors for coronary heart disease: a summary of systematic reviews conducted for the U.S. Preventive Services Task Force. *Ann Intern Med*. 2009;151(7):496-507.

[58] Tzotzas T, Evangelou P, Kiortsis DN. Obesity, weight loss and conditional cardiovascular risk factors. *Obes Rev*. 2011;12(5):e282-9.

[59] Tilg H, Moschen AR. Role of adiponectin and PBEF/visfatin as regulators of inflammation: involvement in obesity-associated diseases. *Clin Sci (Lond)*. 2008;114(4):275-88.

[60] Okamoto Y, Arita Y, Nishida M, et al. An adipocyte-derived plasma protein, adiponectin, adheres to injured vascular walls. *Horm Metab Res*. 2000;32(2):47-50.

[61] Laughlin GA, Barrett-Connor E, May S, Langenberg C. Association of adiponectin with coronary heart disease and mortality: the Rancho Bernardo study. *Am J Epidemiol*. 2007;165(2):164-74.

[62] Wannamethee SG, Whincup PH, Lennon L, Sattar N. Circulating adiponectin levels and mortality in elderly men with and without cardiovascular disease and heart failure. *Arch Intern Med*. 2007;167(14):1510-7.

[63] Pilz S, Mangge H, Wellnitz B, et al. Adiponectin and mortality in patients undergoing coronary angiography. *J Clin Endocrinol Metab*. 2006;91(11):4277-86.

[64] Snijder MB, Heine RJ, Seidell JC, et al. Associations of adiponectin levels with incident impaired glucose metabolism and type 2 diabetes in older men and women: the hoorn study. *Diabetes Care*. 2006;29(11):2498-503.

[65] Bahceci M, Gokalp D, Bahceci S, Tuzcu A, Atmaca S, Arikan S. The correlation between adiposity and adiponectin, tumor necrosis factor alpha, interleukin-6 and high sensitivity C-reactive protein levels. Is adipocyte size associated with inflammation in adults? *J Endocrinol Invest*. 2007;30(3):210-4.

[66] Hotta K, Funahashi T, Arita Y, et al. Plasma concentrations of a novel, adipose-specific protein, adiponectin, in type 2 diabetic patients. *Arterioscler Thromb Vasc Biol*. 2000;20(6):1595-9.

[67] Oh DK, Ciaraldi T, Henry RR. Adiponectin in health and disease. *Diabetes Obes Metab*. 2007;9(3):282-9.

[68] Yang RZ, Lee MJ, Hu H, et al. Identification of omentin as a novel depot-specific adipokine in human adipose tissue: possible role in modulating insulin action. *Am J Physiol Endocrinol Metab*. 2006;290(6):E1253-61.

[69] Zhong X, Li X, Liu F, Tan H, Shang D. Omentin inhibits TNF-alpha-induced expression of adhesion molecules in endothelial cells via ERK/NF-kappaB pathway. *Biochem Biophys Res Commun*. 2012;425(2):401-6.

[70] Auguet T, Quintero Y, Riesco D, et al. New adipokines vaspin and omentin. Circulating levels and gene expression in adipose tissue from morbidly obese women. *BMC Med Genet*. 2011;12:60.

[71] Shibata R, Ouchi N, Takahashi R, et al. Omentin as a novel biomarker of metabolic risk factors. *Diabetol Metab Syndr*. 2012;4(1):37.

[72] Zhong X, Zhang HY, Tan H, et al. Association of serum omentin-1 levels with coronary artery disease. *Acta Pharmacol Sin*. 2011;32(7):873-8.

[73] Gong FY, Zhang SJ, Deng JY, et al. Zinc-alpha2-glycoprotein is involved in regulation of body weight through inhibition of lipogenic enzymes in adipose tissue. *Int J Obes (Lond)*. 2009;33(9):1023-30.

[74] Selva DM, Lecube A, Hernandez C, Baena JA, Fort JM, Simo R. Lower zinc-alpha2-glycoprotein production by adipose tissue and liver in obese patients unrelated to insulin resistance. *J Clin Endocrinol Metab*. 2009;94(11):4499-507.

[75] Bing C, Mracek T, Gao D, Trayhurn P. Zinc-alpha2-glycoprotein: an adipokine modulator of body fat mass? *Int J Obes (Lond)*. 2010;34(11):1559-65.

[76] Leal VO, Lobo JC, Stockler-Pinto MB, et al. Is zinc-alpha2-glycoprotein a cardiovascular protective factor for patients undergoing hemodialysis? *Clin Chim Acta*. 2012;413(5-6):616-9.

[77] Youn BS, Kloting N, Kratzsch J, et al. Serum vaspin concentrations in human obesity and type 2 diabetes. *Diabetes*. 2008;57(2):372-7.

[78] Chang HM, Park HS, Park CY, Song YS, Jang YJ. Association between serum vaspin concentrations and visceral adipose tissue in Korean subjects. *Metabolism*. 2010;59(9):1276-81.

[79] Chang HM, Lee HJ, Park HS, et al. Effects of weight reduction on serum vaspin concentrations in obese subjects: modification by insulin resistance. *Obesity (Silver Spring)*. 2010;18(11):2105-10.

[80] Bluher M. Vaspin in obesity and diabetes: pathophysiological and clinical significance. *Endocrine*. 2012;41(2):176-82.

[81] Bruun JM, Lihn AS, Verdich C, et al. Regulation of adiponectin by adipose tissue-derived cytokines: in vivo and in vitro investigations in humans. *Am J Physiol Endocrinol Metab*. 2003;285(3):E527-33.

[82] Wang B, Trayhurn P. Acute and prolonged effects of TNF-alpha on the expression and secretion of inflammation-related adipokines by human adipocytes differentiated in culture. *Pflugers Arch*. 2006;452(4):418-27.

[83] Sjostrom L, Lindroos AK, Peltonen M, et al. Lifestyle, diabetes, and cardiovascular risk factors 10 years after bariatric surgery. *N Engl J Med*. 2004;351(26):2683-93.

[84] Kulick D, Hark L, Deen D. The bariatric surgery patient: a growing role for registered dietitians. *J Am Diet Assoc*. 2010;110(4):593-9.

[85] Gloy VL, Briel M, Bhatt DL, et al. Bariatric surgery versus non-surgical treatment for obesity: a systematic review and meta-analysis of randomised controlled trials. *BMJ*. 2013;347:f5934.

[86] Santos J, Salgado P, Santos C, et al. Effect of bariatric surgery on weight loss, inflammation, iron metabolism, and lipid profile. *Scand J Surg*. 2014;103(1):21-5.

[87] Parikh MS, Laker S, Weiner M, Hajiseyedjavadi O, Ren CJ. Objective comparison of complications resulting from laparoscopic bariatric procedures. *J Am Coll Surg*. 2006;202(2):252-61.

[88] Flum DR, Belle SH, King WC, et al. Perioperative safety in the longitudinal assessment of bariatric surgery. *N Engl J Med*. 2009;361(5):445-54.

[89] O'Brien PE, MacDonald L, Anderson M, Brennan L, Brown WA. Long-term outcomes after bariatric surgery: fifteen-year follow-up of adjustable gastric banding and a systematic review of the bariatric surgical literature. *Ann Surg*. 2013;257(1):87-94.

[90] Cigdem Arica P, Kocael A, Tabak O, Taskin M, Zengin K, Uzun H. Plasma ghrelin, leptin, and orexin-A levels and insulin resistance after laparoscopic gastric band applications in morbidly obese patients. *Minerva Med*. 2013;104(3):309-16.

[91] Gelisgen R, Zengin K, Kocael A, et al. Effects of laparoscopic gastric band applications on plasma and fundic acylated ghrelin levels in morbidly obese patients. *Obes Surg*. 2012;22(2):299-305.

[92] Caiazzo R, Arnalsteen L, Pigeyre M, et al. Long-term metabolic outcome and quality of life after laparoscopic adjustable gastric banding in obese patients with type 2 diabetes mellitus or impaired fasting glucose. *Br J Surg*. 2010;97(6):884-91.

[93] Himpens J, Cadiere GB, Bazi M, Vouche M, Cadiere B, Dapri G. Long-term outcomes of laparoscopic adjustable gastric banding. *Arch Surg*. 2011;146(7):802-7.

[94] Ray JB, Ray S. Safety, efficacy, and durability of laparoscopic adjustable gastric banding in a single surgeon U.S. community practice. *Surg Obes Relat Dis*. 2011;7(2):140-4.

[95] te Riele WW, Boerma D, Wiezer MJ, Borel Rinkes IH, van Ramshorst B. Long-term results of laparoscopic adjustable gastric banding in patients lost to follow-up. *Br J Surg*. 2010;97(10):1535-40.

[96] Cobourn C, Chapman MA, Ali A, Amrhein J. Five-year weight loss experience of outpatients receiving laparoscopic adjustable gastric band surgery. *Obes Surg*. 2013;23(7):903-10.

[97] Miller K, Pump A, Hell E. Vertical banded gastroplasty versus adjustable gastric banding: prospective long-term follow-up study. *Surg Obes Relat Dis*. 2007;3(1):84-90.

[98] Kasza J, Brody F, Vaziri K, et al. Analysis of poor outcomes after laparoscopic adjustable gastric banding. *Surg Endosc*. 2011;25(1):41-7.

[99] Chakravarty PD, McLaughlin E, Whittaker D, et al. Comparison of laparoscopic adjustable gastric banding (LAGB) with other bariatric procedures; a systematic review of the randomised controlled trials. *Surgeon*. 2012;10(3):172-82.

[100] Pilone V, Mozzi E, Schettino AM, et al. Improvement in health-related quality of life in first year after laparoscopic adjustable gastric banding. *Surg Obes Relat Dis*. 2012;8(3):260-8.

[101] Dixon JB, O'Brien PE, Playfair J, et al. Adjustable gastric banding and conventional therapy for type 2 diabetes: a randomized controlled trial. *JAMA*. 2008;299(3):316-23.

[102] Dixon JB, O'Brien PE. Health outcomes of severely obese type 2 diabetic subjects 1 year after laparoscopic adjustable gastric banding. *Diabetes Care*. 2002;25(2):358-63.

[103] Brancatisano A, Wahlroos S, Matthews S, Brancatisano R. Gastric banding for the treatment of type 2 diabetes mellitus in morbidly obese. *Surg Obes Relat Dis*. 2008;4(3):423-9.

[104] Ritt M, Piza H, Rhomberg M, Aigner F, Lechleitner M. Metabolic risk factors in formerly obese women--effects of a pronounced weight loss by gastric band operation compared with weight loss by diet alone. *Diabetes Obes Metab*. 2005;7(3):216-22.

[105] Sultan S, Gupta D, Parikh M, et al. Five-year outcomes of patients with type 2 diabetes who underwent laparoscopic adjustable gastric banding. *Surg Obes Relat Dis*. 2010;6(4):373-6.

[106] Trakhtenbroit MA, Leichman JG, Algahim MF, et al. Body weight, insulin resistance, and serum adipokine levels 2 years after 2 types of bariatric surgery. *Am J Med*. 2009;122(5):435-42.

[107] Plum L, Ahmed L, Febres G, et al. Comparison of glucostatic parameters after hypocaloric diet or bariatric surgery and equivalent weight loss. *Obesity (Silver Spring)*. 2011;19(11):2149-57.

[108] Bradley D, Conte C, Mittendorfer B, et al. Gastric bypass and banding equally improve insulin sensitivity and beta cell function. *J Clin Invest*. 2012;122(12):4667-74.

[109] Tussing-Humphreys LM, Nemeth E, Fantuzzi G, et al. Decreased serum hepcidin and improved functional iron status 6 months after restrictive bariatric surgery. *Obesity (Silver Spring)*. 2010;18(10):2010-6.

[110] Marantos G, Daskalakis M, Karkavitsas N, Matalliotakis I, Papadakis JA, Melissas J. Changes in metabolic profile and adipoinsular axis in morbidly obese premenopausal females treated with restrictive bariatric surgery. *World J Surg*. 2011;35(9):2022-30.

[111] Ram E, Vishne T, Maayan R, et al. The relationship between BMI, plasma leptin, insulin and proinsulin before and after laparoscopic adjustable gastric banding. *Obes Surg*. 2005;15(10):1456-62.

[112] Shak JR, Roper J, Perez-Perez GI, et al. The effect of laparoscopic gastric banding surgery on plasma levels of appetite-control, insulinotropic, and digestive hormones. *Obes Surg*. 2008;18(9):1089-96.

[113] Moschen AR, Molnar C, Wolf AM, et al. Effects of weight loss induced by bariatric surgery on hepatic adipocytokine expression. *J Hepatol*. 2009;51(4):765-77.

[114] Korner J, Inabnet W, Febres G, et al. Prospective study of gut hormone and metabolic changes after adjustable gastric banding and Roux-en-Y gastric bypass. *Int J Obes (Lond)*. 2009;33(7):786-95.

[115] Krieger AC, Youn H, Modersitzki F, et al. Effects of laparoscopic adjustable gastric banding on sleep and metabolism: a 12-month follow-up study. *Int J Gen Med.* 2012;5:975-81.

[116] Uzun H, Zengin K, Taskin M, Aydin S, Simsek G, Dariyerli N. Changes in leptin, plasminogen activator factor and oxidative stress in morbidly obese patients following open and laparoscopic Swedish adjustable gastric banding. *Obes Surg*. 2004;14(5):659-65.

[117] Botella-Carretero JI, Luque-Ramirez M, Alvarez-Blasco F, Peromingo R, San Millan JL, Escobar-Morreale HF. The increase in serum visfatin after bariatric surgery in morbidly obese women is modulated by weight loss, waist circumference, and presence or absence of diabetes before surgery. *Obes Surg*. 2008;18(8):1000-6.

[118] Garcia-Fuentes E, Garcia-Almeida JM, Garcia-Arnes J, et al. Plasma visfatin concentrations in severely obese subjects are increased after intestinal bypass. *Obesity (Silver Spring)*. 2007;15(10):2391-5.

[119] De Vriese C, Delporte C. Ghrelin: a new peptide regulating growth hormone release and food intake. *Int J Biochem Cell Biol*. 2008;40(8):1420-4.

[120] Tschop M, Weyer C, Tataranni PA, Devanarayan V, Ravussin E, Heiman ML. Circulating ghrelin levels are decreased in human obesity. *Diabetes*. 2001;50(4):707-9.

[121] Hanusch-Enserer U, Cauza E, Brabant G, et al. Plasma ghrelin in obesity before and after weight loss after laparoscopical adjustable gastric banding. *J Clin Endocrinol Metab*. 2004;89(7):3352-8.

[122] Hady HR, Dadan J, Golaszewski P. 100 obese patients after laparoscopic adjustable gastric banding - the influence on BMI, gherlin and insulin concentration, parameters of lipid balance and co-morbidities. *Adv Med Sci*. 2012;57(1):58-64.

[123] Zengin K, Taskin M, Sakoglu N, Salihoglu Z, Demiroluk S, Uzun H. Systemic inflammatory response after laparoscopic and open application of adjustable banding for morbidly obese patients. *Obes Surg*. 2002;12(2):276-9.

[124] Lasselin J, Magne E, Beau C, et al. Adipose inflammation in obesity: relationship with circulating levels of inflammatory markers and association with surgery-induced weight loss. *J Clin Endocrinol Metab*. 2014;99(1):E53-61.

[125] Keogh JB, Brancatisano A, Taylor SF, et al. Evaluation of the Swedish adjustable gastric band VC (SAGB-VC) in an Australian population: early results. *Can J Surg*. 2013;56(1):15-20.

[126] Ramalho R, Guimaraes C, Gil C, Neves C, Guimaraes JT, Delgado L. Morbid obesity and inflammation: a prospective study after adjustable gastric banding surgery. *Obes Surg*. 2009;19(7):915-20.

[127] Cugno M, Castelli R, Mari D, et al. Inflammatory and prothrombotic parameters in normotensive non-diabetic obese women: effect of weight loss obtained by gastric banding. *Intern Emerg Med*. 2012;7(3):237-42.

[128] Moschen AR, Molnar C, Geiger S, et al. Anti-inflammatory effects of excessive weight loss: potent suppression of adipose interleukin 6 and tumour necrosis factor alpha expression. *Gut*. 2010;59(9):1259-64.

[129] Gasteyger C, Suter M, Calmes JM, Gaillard RC, Giusti V. Changes in body composition, metabolic profile and nutritional status 24 months after gastric banding. *Obes Surg*. 2006;16(3):243-50.

[130] Samaras K, Viardot A, Botelho NK, Jenkins A, Lord RV. Immune cell-mediated inflammation and the early improvements in glucose metabolism after gastric banding surgery. *Diabetologia*. 2013;56(12):2564-72.

[131] Tulchinsky TH. Micronutrient deficiency conditions: global health issues. *Publ Health Rev*. 2010;32:243 - 55.

[132] Nead KG, Halterman JS, Kaczorowski JM, Auinger P, Weitzman M. Overweight children and adolescents: a risk group for iron deficiency. *Pediatrics*. 2004;114(1):104-8.

[133] Yanoff LB, Menzie CM, Denkinger B, et al. Inflammation and iron deficiency in the hypoferremia of obesity. *Int J Obes (Lond)*. 2007;31(9):1412-9.

[134] Lecube A, Carrera A, Losada E, Hernandez C, Simo R, Mesa J. Iron deficiency in obese postmenopausal women. *Obesity (Silver Spring)*. 2006;14(10):1724-30.

[135] Zimmermann MB, Zeder C, Muthayya S, et al. Adiposity in women and children from transition countries predicts decreased iron absorption, iron deficiency and a reduced response to iron fortification. *Int J Obes (Lond)*. 2008;32(7):1098-104.

[136] Lee PL, Beutler E. Regulation of hepcidin and iron-overload disease. *Annu Rev Pathol*. 2009;4:489-515.

[137] Nemeth E, Tuttle MS, Powelson J, et al. Hepcidin regulates cellular iron efflux by binding to ferroportin and inducing its internalization. *Science*. 2004;306(5704):2090-3.

[138] Nicolas G, Chauvet C, Viatte L, et al. The gene encoding the iron regulatory peptide hepcidin is regulated by anemia, hypoxia, and inflammation. *J Clin Invest*. 2002;110(7):1037-44.

[139] Collins JF, Wessling-Resnick M, Knutson MD. Hepcidin regulation of iron transport. *J Nutr*. 2008;138(11):2284-8.

[140] Bekri S, Gual P, Anty R, et al. Increased adipose tissue expression of hepcidin in severe obesity is independent from diabetes and NASH. *Gastroenterology*. 2006;131(3): 788-96.

[141] Vokurka M, Lacinova Z, Kremen J, et al. Hepcidin expression in adipose tissue increases during cardiac surgery. *Physiol Res*. 2010;59(3):393-400.

[142] Luciani N, Brasse-Lagnel C, Poli M, et al. Hemojuvelin: a new link between obesity and iron homeostasis. *Obesity (Silver Spring)*. 2011;19(8):1545-51.

[143] Anty R, Dahman M, Iannelli A, et al. Bariatric surgery can correct iron depletion in morbidly obese women: a link with chronic inflammation. *Obes Surg*. 2008;18(6):709-14.

[144] Coupaye M, Bouillot JL, Coussieu C, Guy-Grand B, Basdevant A, Oppert JM. One-year changes in energy expenditure and serum leptin following adjustable gastric banding in obese women. *Obes Surg*. 2005;15(6):827-33.

[145] Diker D, Vishne T, Maayan R, et al. Impact of gastric banding on plasma adiponectin levels. *Obes Surg*. 2006;16(8):1057-61.

[146] Benedix F, Westphal S, Patschke R, et al. Weight loss and changes in salivary ghrelin and adiponectin: comparison between sleeve gastrectomy and Roux-en-Y gastric bypass and gastric banding. *Obes Surg*. 2011;21(5):616-24.

[147] Visockiene Z, Brimas G, Abaliksta T, Siauliene L, Liakina V, Strupas K. Metabolic changes one year after laparoscopic adjustable gastric banding operation in morbidly obese subjects. *Wideochir Inne Tech Malo Inwazyjne*. 2013;8(1):13-21.

In: Bariatric Surgery
Editor: Mandy Chambers

ISBN: 978-1-63463-697-1

Chapter 6

Pregnancy after Bariatric Surgery

Catarina Policiano, Alexandre Valentim Lourenço, Luísa Pinto and Luís Mendes Graça
Department of Obstetrics and Gynecology, University Hospital of Santa Maria,
Centro Hospitalar Lisboa Norte, Lisbon, Portugal

Obesity Epidemic and Its Impact on Pregnancy

Obesity rates and its serious comorbidities have been rising worldwide resulting in a significant loss of life expectancy [1, 2]. Women of reproductive age are generally healthy and metabolic disorders in this age group are uncommon. However they account for a large group of the obese population and pre-pregnancy Body Mass Index (BMI) has been strongly associated with an increased risk of diabetes, hypertension and dyslipidemia, not only during pregnancy but also in the following decades of life. Pre-pregnancy overweight and obesity are also independent risk factors for serious comorbid cardiovascular events (ischemic heart disease, cardiac heart failure) even in the absence of metabolic syndrome [3-5].

The Impact on Fertility

The excess of adipose tissue has been demonstrated to be associated with increased secretion of a wide variety of cytokines and hormone-like factors, such as leptine and acute-phase proteins [6, 7]. The proinflammatory state and the metabolic dysfunction may justify the higher rates of infertility in obese women, particularly in the case of polycystic ovary syndrome (PCOS). The pathophysiology of PCOS is unclear and this entity is commonly defined as oligo- or anovulation, hyperandrogenism, and polycystic ovaries. This condition affects 6-25% of reproductive-age women and at least half of the women with PCOS are obese, representing potential bariatric surgery patients [8].

There are various reports of the negative impact of obesity on the success of assisted-reproductive technology (ART) [9]. Hirshfeld-Cytron et al. described a case of a woman that had been submitted to a gastric bypass with the loss of approximately 79 Kg and who presented for controlled ovarian hyperstimulation, which resulted in an empty follicle syndrome, resolved by changing the route of administration of human chorionic gonadotropin (hCG). The authors hypothesized that in the setting of dramatic weight loss after bariatric surgery, skin redundancy may limit the bioavailability of subcutaneous hCG. This limitation was overtaken by changing the route of administration to intramuscular [10]. Several publications have also discussed the role of weight loss in obese women with infertility, in particular the specific role in improving the rates of conception and live births [11]. Nonetheless, the heterogeneity of the samples and of the outcomes in the published studies resulted in no consensus on the effect of maternal weight on the outcomes of ART [12].

Obesity and Pregnancy

Obesity in pregnancy is defined as a pre-pregnancy BMI $\geq$ 30 Kg/m^2 [13]. BMI is an independent predictive risk factor of maternal-fetal adverse outcomes [14-16]. The recommended total weight gain for overweight (BMI 25-30 Kg/m^2) and obese women is 7.0-11.5 kg and 5.0-9.0 kg, respectively, based on the guidelines of the Institute of Medicine [17]. Extreme obesity (BMI $\geq$ 50 Kg/m^2) imparts a significant increase of obstetric complications such as hypertensive disorders of pregnancy and gestational diabetes, macrosomia, shoulder dystocia, perineal trauma at birth and higher rates of cesarean deliveries, compared to all-other obese and non-obese women. Furthermore, neonates from extremely obese women are more likely to have metabolic disturbances and to be admitted to the Neonatal Intensive Care Unit (NICU) [18-20].

Regarding the higher risk of diabetes, it is generally accepted that the underlying mechanism consists on an exaggerated insulin resistance that is characteristic both of the pregnant and of the obese woman [21].

Obese women are prone to develop metabolic syndrome with all its typical components such as hypertension. Hypertensive disorders including preeclampsia (association between hypertension and proteinuria during pregnancy or in the postpartum period) and eclampsia (preeclampsia with convulsions) are more frequent in the obese population. It is hypothesized that obesity in pregnant women predisposes to preeclampsia due to an up-regulated systemic inflammatory reaction and hyperlipidemia (mark removed) [22, 23].

Obesity: Difficulty of Ultrasound Screening and Risk of Malformations

Obesity in pregnancy poses difficulties in the ultrasonographic diagnosis of fetal anomalies even for experienced sonographers [24]. Images are more difficult to interpret because of abdominal adiposity. A recent report has found higher number of ultrasound evaluations in this population. Among obese women, 48% had five or more ultrasound scans compared to 25% in the nonobese group ($p < 0.05$) [25]. Despite the technical difficulties, literature points out an increased ultrasound detection of specific structural anomalies, such as neural tube defects, cardiovascular, face and limb anomalies, when comparing to average-weight women [26, 27]. Some recent studies in animal models have demonstrated that maternal obesity may not only be associated with lifelong deleterious metabolic effects on the developing child such as all the underlying comorbidities (diabetes, hypertension...space removed) but may also imply future neurologic disorders. The explanation of the investigators relies on alterations on neuronal proliferation, maturation and migration in association with the abnormal hormonal and inflammatory environment characteristic of obesity [28, 29].

Maternal obesity has been associated with increased risk of developing asthma during childhood. Furthermore, children´s overweight is also an important predisposing factor and in both cases the mechanism that justifies the relationship between obesity and asthma seems to be an excess of inflammatory reaction [30].

Obese women have a higher incidence of dizygotic twin gestation when compared to average weight women. The possible explanation for this association relies on the elevated follicle-stimulating hormone levels [31].

A large study from Sweden including 1,599,551 deliveries, demonstrated that maternal overweight and obesity were associated with higher rates of spontaneous and medically indicated preterm deliveries, especially extremely preterm compared to normal weight women. [32]

Regarding the route of delivery, pre-pregnancy obesity imparts a higher risk of cesarean section. A systematic review on the risk for cesarean deliveries in obese nulliparous women demonstrated that the risk for cesarean delivery is increased by 50% in overweight women and is more than double for obese women compared with women with normal BMI [33]. Longer first stage of labor and higher rate of fetal heart rate abnormalities are contributors to the increased rate of cesarean deliveries [34-35]. Moreover, a cesarean section in an obese woman is associated with more frequent perioperative morbidities, such as longer operative times, excessive blood loss, anesthetic difficulties (epidural failure, difficult intubation), infectious and thromboembolic events. Obesity is also associated with short-term perinatal risks of macrosomia, birth trauma and shoulder dystocia [35, 36].

Lifestyle interventions (diet, exercise) in overweight and obese pregnant women give important contributions in reducing maternal complications such as hypertensive disorders, diabetes and shoulder dystocia. It is absolutely essential to encourage weight loss at the pre-conception counseling appointments since it has been proven that the pregravid excess of weight implies a higher risk pregnancy compared to the excessive weight gained during pregnancy. All the comorbidities that have been described above will result in longer hospital stay leading to increased overall healthcare costs compared to average weight women. Unfortunately lifestyle interventions are frequently ineffective in the long-term achievement and maintenance of weight loss. Furthermore, there are no truly effective pharmacological agents to treat obesity, especially morbid obesity [37-38].

Types of Bariatric Surgery: Advantages and Limitations for Pregnant Women

Bariatric surgery is recommended for the treatment of morbid obesity (BMI $\geq 40Kg/m^2$) or class II obesity (BMI $\geq 35Kg/m^2$ with associated co-morbidities) and it is an increasingly selected option for obesity refractory to lifestyle intervention and medical treatment. It is the most effective approach to these situations, resulting in partial or complete resolution of comorbidities associated with obesity and improving the quality of life of the patients. Epidemiological studies report that women of reproductive age account for about half of the patients that have been submitted to bariatric surgery [39, 40].

Bariatric surgery comprises two major types of surgeries according to the main mechanism of weight loss: restrictive or malabsorptive. Restrictive procedures, such as adjustable gastric band, contribute to the limiting of caloric intake by reducing gastric volume, implying only mild nutritional deficiencies. Malabsorptive surgeries, such as biliopancreatic diversion, induce weight loss by generating an asynergy between the bolus and the biliopancreatic secretions, subsequently implying a higher protein and micronutrients (iron, calcium, vitamin B12, folate and vitamin D) deficiency compared to exclusively restrictive procedures. Gastric bypass, the most common weight loss surgery performed worldwide, is a technique that comprises both mechanisms of weight loss but is predominantly malabsorptive. Comparing the two most commonly used methods, laparoscopic adjustable gastric banding and Roux-en-Y gastric bypass, the last one is considered the most effective in terms of weight loss. Despite the longer operative time and the higher rate of perioperative morbidity associated with gastric bypass, in the long-term follow up, gastric banding requires more frequently reoperation. The majority of bariatric surgeries may be performed by laparoscopy with safer and less invasive procedures [41].

In nonpregnant obese patients, bariatric surgery contributes to reverse, eliminate or to improve many serious comorbid illnesses of the metabolic syndrome, such as impaired glucose tolerance, dyslipidemia and hypertension, leading in the long-term to an increase in life expectancy by decreasing the related deaths due to cardiovascular disease and complications. According to Buchwald et al., more than three quarters of patients with type 2 diabetes experience complete resolution of the disease after bariatric surgery. Of those patients who fail to achieve complete resolution, more than half showed demonstrable improvement. Thus, about 85% of patients with diabetes experienced improvement in their diabetes evolution after bariatric surgery [42]. Other medical conditions caused or aggravated by obesity, such as sleep apnea, daytime sleepiness, asthma, and gastroesophageal reflux are also significantly improved by the weight reduction after bariatric surgery. Moreover there is significant improvement in the quality of life and psychosocial wellbeing of morbidly obese patients [43]. Hormonal and mechanical factors of pregnancy alter the structure and function of the normal physiological barriers to reflux of gastric contents into the esophagus, and overweight is an aggravating factor that predisposes to complaints refractory to lifestyle and medical treatment. Thus, bariatric surgery as an effective promoter of weight reduction contributes to avoid the aggravating effect of obesity in physiological changes that are characteristic of pregnancy and otherwise would be symptomatic and difficult to control.

Several studies report an important improvement in fertility after bariatric surgery, particularly in hyperandrogenic and anovulatory women, independently of the type of bariatric surgery [40].

Potential complications such as micronutrient deficiencies are more commonly associated with malabsorptive surgery than with restrictive bariatric surgery. Restrictive procedures such as adjustable gastric band may be loosened during pregnancy permitting the individualization of caloric and gastric volume reduction. These surgeries are also less frequently responsible for late surgical complications than predominantly malabsorptive surgeries, such as gastric bypass. The band consists of an inflatable balloon whose diameter can be adjusted in ambulatory care by adding or removing saline solution via a reservoir port positioned beneath the skin. The bands are adjustable to allow the size of the gastric outlet to be modified as needed in order to be adequate for gestational age weight gain. There are no randomized trials comparing elective deflation versus indicated deflation of the gastric band during pregnancy in terms of maternal-fetal outcomes. A recent retrospective study suggested that band loosening should be reserved for symptomatic patients in order to avoid excessive weight gain [44].

Pregnancy should be postponed until at least 12 to 18 months after bariatric surgery in an attempt to avoid the theoretical potential adverse effect of the intense nutritional deficiencies that may affect both fetus and mother during the rapid weight loss phase. If this vulnerable time period coincides with the time of elevated nutritional needs of a pregnancy, some reports highlight the possibility of a malnourished fetus and of potential complications such as low birth weight and malformations [45, 46]. Despite the inconsistent scientific evidence that supports the need to postpone pregnancy for a specific period after bariatric surgery and the lack of randomized trials showing significant differences in maternal-fetal morbidity and mortality, a recent retrospective cohort study, that compared pregnancy outcomes between women who conceived less than two years and more than two years after bariatric surgery, found that in the first group there were higher rates of gestational diabetes and lower weight loss [46]. Nonetheless, in case of pregnancy in the first year after surgery, women should be reassured that there is no scientific evidence of increased adverse neonatal outcomes. [47].

The American College of Obstetricians and Gynecologists (ACOG) recommends effective non-oral contraception, especially in women that have undergone malabsorptive surgery and do not pretend or have formal contraindications to get pregnant [48]. Oral contraception, especially after malabsorptive surgeries, may suffer a limited and irregular absorption leading to unreliable pharmacological effectiveness.

Regarding anatomic gastrointestinal complications, data from several reports suggest that they are more frequently associated with malbsorptive surgeries such as gastric bypass. Dumping syndrome consists on the effect of fast absorption carbohydrates that are rapidly emptied into the small bowel causing an osmotic shift of excessive fluid from the intravascular compartment to the small bowel lumen. This will cause abdominal cramping, bloating, nausea, vomiting and diarrhea. Symptoms of tachycardia, palpitations, anxiety and diaphoresis may be due not only to intravascular depletion but also to the secondary hypersecretion of insulin, which results in hypoglycemia. As a result, patients develop an aversion to high-carbohydrate foods, which leads to major changes in their diet and eating habits. Pregnant women submitted to bariatric surgery usually do not tolerate the standard oral glucose tolerance test for screening of gestational diabetes. An alternative method that has been suggested includes the outpatient evaluation of fasting capillary blood glucose and a 2-hour postprandial sample for 1 week between 24-28 weeks of gestation (the gestational age recommended for the standard evaluation). Women with previous restrictive surgeries, such as adjustable gastric band, rarely develop dumping syndrome and usually tolerate the standard glucose challenge test [48].

Understanding the underlying mechanism of each type of bariatric surgery is critical for an adequate counseling of patients. Pregnancy after bariatric surgery is associated with significant decreased rates of hypertensive disorders and gestational diabetes as well as lower rates of fetal macrosomia, comparing to obese women who have not undergone bariatric surgery [47].

Concise guidelines for counseling and management of reproductive-aged women that have undergone bariatric surgery are lacking. Moreover, there is neither consensus on the adequate management of pregnant women previously submitted to bariatric surgery nor specific recommendations on the role of the bariatric surgeon. Nonetheless, several international societies and committees recommend tight monitoring of maternal nutrition and vitamin supplementation as well as close supervision with the collaboration of the bariatric surgeon and nutritionist [48].

Nutritional Deficiencies

As mentioned above, nutritional derangements can occur after bariatric surgery. These are particularly severe and frequent after malaborptive procedures. Macronutrient deficiencies such as protein–calorie malnutrition and fat malabsorption, deficiencies in fat-soluble vitamins in association with deficit of several micronutrients and minerals, particularly iron, folate, vitamin B12, vitamin D and calcium may occur after gastric bypass. Absorption of iron and folate are diminished because of reduced availability of acid in the gastric pouch and also due to the bypass of the duodenum, the major site for the absorption of these two micronutrients [40, 42].

Patients with morbid obesity (usually the population submitted to bariatric surgery) may develop secondary hyperparathyroidism and vitamin D deficiency. The abrupt weight loss imparted by bariatric surgery is frequently accompanied by the regression of secondary hyperparathyroidism and the improvement of vitamin D deficiency and bone turnover. Dietary calcium is mainly absorbed in the duodenum. After Roux-en-Y gastric bypass, food stream bypasses the majority of the stomach and duodenum, causing chronic calcium deficiency which may result in secondary hyperparathyroidism and vitamin D deficiency, counteracting the improvement caused by weight loss. There are reports of osteopenia and metabolic bone disease after bariatric malabsorptive surgery. Supplementation with vitamin D and calcium is recommended in these cases [49].

Absorption of food vitamin B12 occurs in the terminal ileum. However the absorption requires an adequate gastric acid secretion and the prior combination with intrinsic factor, which is produced in the gastric mucosa, and may be deficient in women previously submitted to gastric bypass.

Laparoscopic adjustable gastric band has been only associated with folate deficiency. The importance of normal levels in prenatal and first trimester assessments in order to avoid neural tube defects makes it fundamental to routinely monitor the levels of folate before and during pregnancy.

The absence of an adequate multivitamin supplementation may have important negative consequences for the fetus such as: cerebral hemorrhages due to vitamin K deficiency; microcephaly, hypotonia, microphthalmia and permanent retinal damage due to vitamin A deficiency; anemia due to vitamin B12 and iron deficiency and fetal deaths [50].

Pregnant women previously submitted to a bariatric operation should have a nutritional assessment preconception and during pregnancy for deficiencies of micronutrients. There is no consensus on the adequate nutritional supplementation during pregnancy and the daily doses are mainly extrapolated from observational studies and expert opinions. Vitamin B12 storage is enough for about 12 to 18 months. If replacement is needed, a daily oral dose of

500 mcg is recommended. However the lack of intrinsic factor may prevent intestinal absorption and weekly intramuscular injections of 1000 mcg are usually more effective. In order to prevent anemia and neural tube defects, Beard et al. recommend that folate (400 mcg) and iron (50-100 mg daily) should be routinely supplemented during pregnancy. Furthermore, at least 1,000 mg calcium (maximum of 1,500 mg) is also recommended [50]. Vitamin A supplementation should be limited to 5000 IU per day in order to avoid retinoid embryopathy [48].

Nutritional monitoring should continue in puerperal women who are breastfeeding [48].

High restriction of the daily intake of calories or proteins is not recommended in the case of pregnancy after bariatric surgery, even if there is persistence of a high BMI, because caloric restriction may impair fetal growth.

Maternal-Fetal Outcomes after Bariatric Surgery

Despite the lack of rigorous randomized studies, pregnant women who have been submitted to bariatric surgery have lower rates of many adverse maternal and neonatal outcomes compared to pregnant women who are obese without bariatric surgery and pregnancy outcome is similar to that in the general population [47].

Pregnancy after Malabsorptive VS after Restrictive Surgeries

Pregnancy after gastric bypass is more consistently reported in the literature in association with serious complications such as bowel obstruction, dumping syndrome, hemorrhage and herniation compared to restrictive surgeries. Gastrointestinal complaints may mimic non-specific symptoms of pregnancy such as hyperemesis, esophageal reflux and uterine contractions, requiring a high index of suspicion in order to disclose them. Misdiagnosis or delayed diagnosis may lead to maternal morbidity and mortality. Recently, a cohort study showed an incidence of 1% of internal herniation during pregnancy, which is a potentially serious complication that requires immediate surgical intervention even in the absence of typical findings on imaging exams [51]. The enlarging gravid uterus imposes an increased abdominal pressure and cephalad displacement of the bowel, contributing to herniation, obstruction, potentially life-threatening bowel strangulation and sepsis, which may be lethal to both mother and fetus [47].

Gastrointestinal complications in pregnant women with previous insertion of a gastric band are rarer than after gastric bypass but some serious complications such as gastric ulceration, band erosion and slippage have been reported in the literature. [52-54].

Pregnancy increases the risk of gallstone disease due to decreased gallbladder emptying and motility as well as changes in the chemical components of bile (increased cholesterol saturation and decreased bile acid content). Acute cholecystitis is the second most common nonobstetrical surgical emergency during pregnancy, after acute appendicitis. The frequency of symptomatic gallstones after malabsorptive surgery is significantly higher than after restrictive procedures. This difference has been attributed to the rapid weight loss after malabsorptive techniques, which is thought to be an important factor in inducing gallstones formation postoperatively. Thus, the occurrence of pregnancy during the postoperative period of maximum weight loss is an additional risk factor for cholelithiasis and its complications, such as cholecystitis and pancreatitis [55].

Fetal Outcomes after Bariatric Surgery

Obese pregnant women have higher rates of extremes of growth disorders – low birth weight and macrosomia –, probably due to higher rates of vascular complications and gestational diabetes, respectively. After bariatric surgery, all the metabolic changes related to nutritional deficiencies impart a decrease in the mean birth weight, consequently decreasing the rate of macrosomia and increasing the number of small for gestational age neonates compared not only to obese women without bariatric surgery but also in comparison to the general population [56]. Weintraub et al. compared pre- and post-bariatric pregnancies and reported more than 50 percent decrease in the risk of macrosomia [57]. Regarding the rate of fetal growth restriction there is no consensus in the literature. The role of nutritional deficiency as an important risk factor that may induce poor fetal growth may be balanced by the decreased risk of preeclampsia after bariatric surgery that may account for lower cases of fetal growth restriction in this context.

Fetal adverse outcomes include the risk of small for gestation age due to chronic nutrient malabsorption as well as the acute metabolic consequences of maternal fasting in case of prolonged symptoms of gastrointestinal obstruction. We have recently reported a clinical case of gastric rupture finding during a cesarean section in a woman with an adjustable gastric band [58]. Despite the obvious maternal morbidity with the need of partial gastrectomy, we discussed the fetal repercussion of the hemoperitoneum from gastric rupture as well as the effect of prolonged maternal fasting and metabolic acidosis. The poor nutritional status of the mother can be exacerbated by vomiting or nausea during pregnancy. When inadequately corrected during pregnancy, serious health problems may occur in the fetus, such as growth retardation and electrolyte imbalances. Probably too restrictive bariatric surgeries with an exaggerated limitation of nutrient intake would result in maternal malnutrition or starvation. Consequently the accumulation of ketone bodies would condition in extreme situation a fasting acidemia. It is still not known the exact effect of maternal acidemia on fetal acid base balance.

Multidisciplinary management of pregnancy with an active role of the bariatric surgeon is essential to disclose the need for immediate surgical intervention. Adjustable gastric band is a reversible bariatric surgery and deflation is a possible solution for women with gastric obstruction symptoms. It is absolutely essential to evaluate the effectiveness of this intervention and if symptoms persist after removal of fluid of the band it may suggest band slippage or gastric prolapse. With these suspicions surgical exploration should be a first option. Imaging exams should not be avoided with the fear of fetal harm, since the correct diagnosis of an obstruction or herniation may prevent fetal morbidity and death. Case reports of maternal deaths have been described in the literature, mainly due to a delayed diagnosis [59, 60].

Previous bariatric surgery is not an indication for the anticipation of delivery or for a cesarean section and both decisions should be made in accordance with standard obstetric criteria [48]. The increased rate of cesarean deliveries in some observational studies of pregnant women after bariatric surgery is associated with obesity, gastrointestinal complications and medically indicated preterm delivery [61]. The bariatric surgery is not an established independent risk factor for cesarean section [56].

There is no evidence of increased delivery complications in pregnancy after bariatric surgery, such as low Apgar scores, meconium-stained amniotic fluid, NICU admission, perinatal mortality rate, congenital malformations. Moreover, there is also no difference in neonatal outcomes between malabsorptive and restrictive surgeries [62].

Conclusion

Prepregnancy obesity is a significant and independent risk factor for both adverse maternal and perinatal outcomes with an increased risk for gestational hypertensive disorders and diabetes. The combination of pregestational metabolic syndrome with the physiological changes of pregnancy imparts an increased risk for maternal disease such as chronic cardiac dysfunction. During labor, obesity increases the risk for cesarean delivery and the associated complications of anesthesia, infection, wound disruption and thromboembolism.

Diet, behavioral therapy, exercise and pharmacological treatment usually yield only modest results and weight loss is frequently regained in a short to medium period of time. Bariatric surgery is a promising treatment for morbidly obese women or in case of failure of lifestyle interventions and medical treatment. Weight loss after these surgeries is associated with an increase in fertility for obese women of reproductive age, especially if there is an anovulatory dysfunction. Pregnancy after bariatric surgery is safe and women are not at increased risk for adverse maternal and perinatal outcomes. Moreover, the major risks for many obesity-related gestational complications are decreased, especially the development of hypertensive disorders and gestational diabetes, as long as appropriate monitoring, nutritional control and efficient prenatal care are provided. Non-oral contraception is recommended during the period of maximum postoperative weight loss (12-18 months) in order to avoid potential risks of complications secondary to poor maternal nutritional status during this period. The most common pregnancy complications after bariatric surgery are nutritional deficiencies, which are easily treated with adequate supplementation. Multidisciplinary surveillance with the collaboration of bariatric surgeon, nutritionist and close obstetrical monitoring are needed to an early detection of any maternal or fetal complications related to previous bariatric surgery. Both obstetricians and surgeons have to consider these pregnant women as high-risk pregnancies, with the need of special care for nutritional assessment and supplementation, and monitoring for adequate weight management.

It is crucial for the obstetrician to know specifically which bariatric procedure the pregnant women had undergone in order to effectively make preconception counseling as well as to prevent and manage potential complications. Malabsorptive interventions impart higher nutritional deficiencies and more frequently are associated with gastrointestinal complications while restrictive procedures such as gastric banding are reversible and adaptable during pregnancy and may be loosened and adjusted to facilitate adequate gestational weight gain. Gastrointestinal complications during pregnancy after bariatric surgery may have only mild and nonspecific symptoms and may also overlap with common obstetric complaints. Late recognition may be life-threatening for both the mother and fetus.

In conclusion, pregnancy in women previously submitted to bariatric surgery is usually safe for the mother and the fetus provided that there is an adequate collaboration between high-risk obstetrician and bariatric surgeon.

References

[1] Pi-Sunyer F. X. The obesity epidemic: Pathophysiology and consequences of obesity. *Obes Res.* 2002; 10:97-104.

[2] National Task Force on the Prevention and Treatment of Obesity. Overweight, obesity, and health risk. *Arch Intern Med.* 2000; 160:898-904.

[3] Schmiegelow M. D., Andersson C., Køber L., Andersen S. S., Norgaard M. L., Jensen T. B., Gislason G., Berger S. M., Torp-Pedersen C. Associations between body mass index and development of metabolic disorders in fertile women: A nationwide cohort study. *J Am Heart Assoc.* 2014. doi: 10.1161/JAHA.113.000672.

[4] Schmiegelow M. D., Andersson C., Køber L., Andersen S. S., Olesen J. B., Jensen T. B., Azimi A., Nielsen M. B., Gislason G., Torp-Pedersen C. Prepregnancy obesity and associations with stroke and myocardial infarction in women in the years after childbirth: a nationwide cohort study. *Circulation.* 2014; 129:330-7.

[5] Thomsen M., Nordestgaard B. G. Myocardial infarction and ischemic heart disease in overweight and obesity with and without metabolic syndrome. *JAMA Intern Med.* 2014; 174:15-22.

[6] Calabrò P., Golia E., Maddaloni V., Malvezzi M., Casillo B., Marotta C., Calabrò R., Golino P. Adipose tissue-mediated inflammation: The missing link between obesity and cardiovascular disease? *Intern Emerg Med.* 2009; 4:25-34.

[7] Calabro P., Yeh E. T. Obesity, inflammation, and vascular disease: The role of the adipose tissue as an endocrine organ. *Subcell Biochem.* 2007; 42:63-91.

[8] Setji T. L., Brown A. J. Polycystic ovary syndrome: update on diagnosis and treatment. *Am J Med.* 2014. doi: 10.1016/j.amjmed.2014.04.017.

[9] Moragianni V. A., Jones S. M., Ryley D. A. The effect of body mass index on the outcomes of first assisted reproductive technology cycles. *Fertil Steril.* 2012; 98:102-8.

[10] Hirshfeld-Cytron J., Kim H. H. Empty follicle syndrome in the setting of dramatic weight loss after bariatric surgery: case report and review of available literature. *Fertil Steril.* 2008; 90:1199.e21-3.

[11] Kort J. D., Winget C., Kim S. H., Lathi R. B. A retrospective cohort study to evaluate the impact of meaningful weight loss on fertility outcomes in an overweight population with infertility. *Fertil Steril.* 2014. doi: 10.1016/j.fertnstert.2014.01.036.

[12] Maheshwari A., Stofberg L., Bhattacharya S. Effect of overweight and obesity on assisted reproductive technology: A systematic review. *Hum Reprod Update.* 2007; 13:433-44.

[13] American College of Obstetricians and Gynecologists. ACOG Committee opinion no. 549: Obesity in pregnancy. *Obstet Gynecol.* 2013; 121:213-7.

[14] Chung J. H., Melsop K. A., Gilbert W. M., Caughey A. B., Walker C. K., Main E. K. Increasing prepregnancy body mass index is predictive of a progressive escalation in adverse pregnancy outcomes. *J Matern Fetal Neonatal Med.* 2012; 25:1635-9.

[15] Crane J. M., White J., Murphy P., Burrage L., Hutchens D. The effect of gestational weight gain by body mass index on maternal and neonatal outcomes. *J Obstet Gynaecol Can.* 2009; 31:28-35.

[16] Scott-Pillai R., Spence D., Cardwell C. R., Hunter A., Holmes V. A. The impact of body mass index on maternal and neonatal outcomes: a retrospective study in a UK obstetric population, 2004-2011. *BJOG.* 2013; 120:932-9.

[17] Rasmussen Z. M., Yaktine A. L. *Weight gain during pregnancy: Reexamining the guidelines.* Institute of Medicine, National Academy of Sciences, National Academies Press, Washington, 2009.

[18] Alanis M. C., Goodnight W. H., Hill E. G., Robinson C. J., Villers M. S., Johnson D. D. Maternal super-obesity (body mass index > or = 50) and adverse pregnancy outcomes. *Acta Obstet Gynecol Scand.* 2010; 89:924-30.

[19] Crane J. M., Murphy P., Burrage L., Hutchens D. Maternal and perinatal outcomes of extreme obesity in pregnancy. *J Obstet Gynaecol Can.* 2013; 35:606-11.

[20] Blomberg M. Maternal obesity, mode of delivery, and neonatal outcome. *Obstet Gynecol.* 2013; 122:50-5.

[21] Catalano P. M., Kirwan J. P., Haugel-de Mouzon S., King J. Gestational diabetes and insulin resistance: role in short- and long-term implications for mother and fetus. *J Nutr.* 2003; 133:1674-83.

[22] Bodnar L. M., Ness R. B., Harger G. F., Roberts J. M. Inflammation and triglycerides partially mediate the effect of prepregnancy body mass index on the risk of preeclampsia. *Am J Epidemiol.* 2005; 162:1198-206.

[23] Rebelo F., Schlüssel M. M., Vaz J. S., Franco-Sena A. B., Pinto T. J., Bastos F. I., Adegboye A. R., Kac G. C-reactive protein and later preeclampsia: Systematic review and meta-analysis taking into account the weight status. *J Hypertens.* 2013; 31:16-26.

[24] Chung J. H., Pelayo R., Hatfield T. J., Speir V. J., Wu J., Caughey A. B. Limitations of the fetal anatomic survey via ultrasound in the obese obstetrical population. *J Matern Fetal Neonatal Med.* 2012; 25:1945-9.

[25] Zozzaro-Smith P., Bacak S., Park J., Spall M., Glantz J. C., Thornburg L. L. Association between obesity during pregnancy and the use of prenatal services. *Obstet Gynecol.* 2014; 123 Suppl 1:80S. doi: 10.1097/01.AOG.0000447404.93680.48.

[26] Stothard K. J., Tennant P. W., Bell R., Rankin J. Stothard K. J., Tennant P. W., Bell R., Rankin J. Maternal overweight and obesity and the risk of congenital anomalies: A systematic review and meta-analysis. *JAMA.* 2009; 301:636-50.

[27] Waller D. K., Shaw G. M., Rasmussen S. A., Hobbs C. A., Canfield M. A., Siega-Riz A. M., Gallaway M. S., Correa A.; National Birth Defects Prevention Study. Prepregnancy obesity as a risk factor for structural birth defects. *Arch Pediatr Adolesc Med.* 2007; 161:745-50.

[28] Stachowiak E. K., Oommen S., Vasu V. T., Srinivasan M., Stachowiak M., Gohil K., Patel M. S. Maternal obesity affects gene expression and cellular development in fetal brains. *Nutr Neurosci.* 2013; 16:96-103.

[29] Stachowiak E. K., Srinivasan M., Stachowiak M. K., Patel M. S. Maternal obesity induced by a high fat diet causes altered cellular development in fetal brains suggestive

of a predisposition of offspring to neurological disorders in later life. *Metab Brain Dis.* 2013; 28:721-5.

[30] Ekström S., Magnusson J., Kull I., Lind T., Almqvist C., Melén E., Bergström A. Maternal BMI in early pregnancy and offspring asthma, rhinitis and eczema up to 16 years of age. *Clin Exp Allergy.* 2014. doi: 10.1111/cea.12340.

[31] Reddy U. M., Branum A. M., Klebanoff M. A. Relationship of maternal body mass index and height to twinning. *Obstet Gynecol.* 2005; 105: 593-7.

[32] Cnattingius S., Villamor E., Johansson S., Edstedt Bonamy A. K., Persson M., Wikström A. K., Granath F. Maternal obesity and risk of preterm delivery. *JAMA.* 2013; 309:2362-70.

[33] Poobalan A. S., Aucott L. S., Gurung T., Smith W. C., Bhattacharya S. Obesity as an independent risk factor for elective and emergency caesarean delivery in nulliparous women--systematic review and meta-analysis of cohort studies. *Obes Rev.* 2009; 10:28-35.

[34] Norman S. M., Tuuli M. G., Odibo A. O., Caughey A. B., Roehl K. A., Cahill A. G. The effects of obesity on the first stage of labor. *Obstet Gynecol.* 2012; 120:130-5.

[35] Chauhan S. P., Magann E. F., Carroll C. S., Barrilleaux P. S., Scardo J. A., Martin J. N Jr. Mode of delivery for the morbidly obese with prior cesarean delivery: Vaginal versus repeat cesarean section. *Am J Obstet Gynecol.* 2001; 185:349-54.

[36] Perlow J. H., Morgan M. A. Massive maternal obesity and perioperative cesarean morbidity. *Am J Obstet Gynecol.* 1994; 170:560-5.

[37] Thangaratinam S., Rogozińska E., Jolly K., Glinkowski S., Duda W., Borowiack E., Roseboom T., Tomlinson J., Walczak J., Kunz R., Mol B. W., Coomarasamy A., Khan K. S. Interventions to reduce or prevent obesity in pregnant women: A systematic review. *Health Technol Assess.* 2012; 16:1-191.

[38] Oteng-Ntim E., Varma R., Croker H., Poston L., Doyle P. Lifestyle interventions for overweight and obese pregnant women to improve pregnancy outcome: Systematic review and meta-analysis. *BMC Med.* 2012; 10:47. doi: 10.1186/1741-7015-10-47.

[39] Santry H. P., Gillen D. L., Lauderdale D. S. Trends in bariatric surgical procedures. *JAMA.* 2005; 294:1909-17.

[40] Shekelle P. G., Newberry S., Maglione M., Li Z., Yermilov I., Hilton L., Suttorp M., Maggard M., Carter J., Tringale C., Chen S. Bariatric surgery in women of reproductive age: special concerns for pregnancy. *Evid Rep Technol Assess* (Full Rep). 2008; 169:1-51.

[41] Tice J. A., Karliner L., Walsh J., Petersen A. J., Feldman M. D. Gastric banding or bypass? A systematic review comparing the two most popular bariatric procedures. *Am J Med.* 2008; 121:885-93.

[42] Buchwald H., Avidor Y., Braunwald E., Jensen M. D., Pories W., Fahrbach K., Schoelles K. Bariatric surgery: A systematic review and meta-analysis. *JAMA.* 2004; 292:1724-37.

[43] Brancatisano A., Wahlroos S., Brancatisano R. Improvement in comorbid illness after placement of the Swedish Adjustable Gastric Band. *Surg Obes Relat Dis.* 2008; 4:S39-46.

[44] Pilone V., Hasani A., di Micco R., Vitiello A., Monda A., Izzo G., Iacobelli L., Villamaina E., Forestieri P. Pregnancy after laparoscopic gastric banding: Maternal and neonatal outcomes. *Int J Surg.* 2014. doi: 10.1016/j.ijsu.2014.05.027.

[45] Magdaleno R. Jr., Pereira B. G., Chaim E. A., Turato E. R. Pregnancy after bariatric surgery: A current view of maternal, obstetrical and perinatal challenges. *Arch Gynecol Obstet.* 2012; 285:559-66.

[46] Parikh R., Lavoie M., Wilson L., Maranda L., Leung K., Simas T. M. Timing of pregnancy after bariatric surgery. *Obstet Gynecol.* 2014; 123. doi: 10.1097/01.AOG. 0000447168.75769.f7.

[47] Kjaer M. M., Nilas L. Pregnancy after bariatric surgery: A review of benefits and risks. *Acta Obstet Gynecol Scand.* 2013; 92:264-71.

[48] American College of Obstetricians and Gynecologists. ACOG practice bulletin no. 105: Bariatric surgery and pregnancy. *Obstet Gynecol.* 2009; 113:1405-13.

[49] De Prisco C., Levine S. N. Metabolic bone disease after gastric bypass surgery for obesity. *Am J Med Sci.* 2005; 329:57-61.

[50] Beard J. H., Bell R. L., Duffy A. J. Reproductive considerations and pregnancy after bariatric surgery: Current evidence and recommendations. *Obes Surg.* 2008; 18:1023-7.

[51] Andreasen L. A., Nilas L., Kjær M. M. Operative Complications during Pregnancy after Gastric Bypass: A Register-Based Cohort Study. *Obes Surg.* 2014 Mar 23 Epub ahead of print.

[52] Suffee M. T., Poncelet C., Barrat C. Gastric band slippage at 30 weeks' gestation: Diagnosis and laparoscopic management. *Surg Obes Relat Dis.* 2012; 8:366-8.

[53] De Nino W. F., Zubarik R. S., Forgione P. M. Laparoscopic gastric band slippage diagnosed with esophagogastroduodenoscopy in a 12-week gestation nulliparous patient. *Surg Obes Relat Dis.* 2011; 7:225-6.

[54] Erez O., Maymon E., Mazor M. Acute gastric ulcer perforation in a 35 weeks' nulliparous patient with gastric banding. *Am J Obstet Gynecol.* 2004; 191:1721-2.

[55] Moon R. C., Teixeira A. F., DuCoin C., Varnadore S., Jawad M. A. Comparison of cholecystectomy cases after Roux-en-Y gastric bypass, sleeve gastrectomy, and gastric banding. *Surg Obes Relat Dis.* 2014; 10:64-8.

[56] Kjær M. M., Lauenborg J., Breum B. M., Nilas L. The risk of adverse pregnancy outcome after bariatric surgery: a nationwide register-based matched cohort study. *Am J Obstet Gynecol.* 2013; 208:464.e1-5.

[57] Weintraub A. Y., Levy A., Levi I., Mazor M., Wiznitzer A., Sheiner E. Effect of bariatric surgery on pregnancy outcome. *Int J Gynaecol Obstet.* 2008; 103:246-51.

[58] Policiano C., Rocha P., Catanho M. C., Pinto L., Valentim-Lourenço A., Graça L. M. Acute fetal asphyxia after gastric rupture in a pregnant patient with a gastric band. *Acta Obstet Gynecol Scand.* 2013; 92:1419-21.

[59] Loar P. V. 3rd, Sanchez-Ramos L., Kaunitz A. M., Kerwin A. J., Diaz J. Maternal death caused by midgut volvulus after bariatric surgery. *Am J Obstet Gynecol.* 2005; 193:1748-9.

[60] Moore K. A., Ouyang D. W., Whang E. E. Maternal and fetal deaths after gastric bypass surgery for morbid obesity. *N Engl J Med.* 2004; 351:721-2.

[61] Roos N., Neovius M., Cnattingius S., Trolle Lagerros Y., Sääf M., Granath F., Stephansson O. Perinatal outcomes after bariatric surgery: Nationwide population based matched cohort study. *BMJ.* 2013; 347: doi: 10.1136/bmj.f6460.

[62] Ducarme G., Parisio L., Santulli P., Carbillon L., Mandelbrot L., Luton D. Neonatal outcomes in pregnancies after bariatric surgery: A retrospective multi-centric cohort study in three French referral centers. *J Matern Fetal Neonatal Med.* 2013; 26:275-8.

In: Bariatric Surgery
Editor: Mandy Chambers

ISBN: 978-1-63463-697-1

Chapter 7

Anesthesia Consideration and Management for Bariatric Surgery

Antoni Sabaté, MD, PhD, DEEA[1]* and Sandra Llaurado, MD[2]
[1]Department of Anesthesia, Reanimation and Pain Clinic, Hospital Universitari de Bellvitge, Universitat de Barcelona Health Campus, Hospitalet, Barcelona, Spain
[2]Department of Anesthesia, Reanimation and Pain Clinic, Hospital Universitari de Bellvitge, Universitat de Barcelona Health Campus, Hospitalet, Barcelona, Spain

Abstract

Morbidly obese patients are already at high risk for cardiovascular and respiratory functional overload related to varying degrees of metabolic syndrome. Most of patients request for bariatric surgery in an early stage of the disease, therefore low rates of mortality and morbidity are the standard. Even that, perioperative complications are related to previous comorbidity, age, body mass index and type of bariatric surgery. Restrictive procedures are not expected to have mortality, but all complication rates are 3.2%, and readmission rate is 4.3%. For gastric bypass procedures, the complication rate is 16%, the readmission rate of 6.6% and mortality around 0.4%, which account intra operatively in 0.18%. of patients. Consequently, anesthetic management of morbid obese patients is a challenge, even to an experienced anesthesiologist and to do that effectively, these key points have to be considered:

Abbreviations

BMI: body mass index
OSA:obstructive sleep apnea
TOFr: the train of four stimulus ratio

* Phone: 34-3-260 7323. Fax: 34-3-260 7998. Correspondence: asabatep@bellvitgehospital.cat, asabatep@ub.edu

1. Safety in Airway Procurement at Anesthesia Induction

In order to facilitate oxygenation and the airway management, patients are placed in semi-sitting position and oxygen is administered to increase tolerance to apnea.

Because neck fat accumulation, difficult tracheal intubation is present in around 10% of patients.

Awake intubation is indicated when a limited mandible advancement is associated to a short tyromental distance [< 6 cm] and a Mallampati class 2/3/4. This conservative approach try to reduce the "can ventilate and can't intubate" crisis, noticed in a range of 0.3-1.2% of patients.

Awake tracheal intubation with videolaringoscope is a good alternative to fiber optical intubation. The introduction of sugammadex, which is able to quickly reverse a neuromuscular blockade of any depth and ensure complete recovery of pharyngeal muscles, have displaced the use of succinylcholine for the patients in whom a general anesthesia induction is planned.

2. Maintenance of Anesthesia during Laparoscopic Procedures

In laparoscopic surgery a deep neuromuscular blockade facilitates ventilation and ensures an adequate surgical field. From a clinical point of view, although neuromuscular monitoring is not widely used, it is therefore advisable. In relation to ventilation strategies during surgery, there is some evidence that recruitment maneuvers added to positive expiratory pressure improved intraoperative oxygenation; but, there is no evidence of any difference between modes of ventilation. Both, desflurane and sevoflurane are suitable for maintenance of anesthesia, and patients are fully awake in a few minutes after switched off the vaporizer. Moreover, both reversal of neuromuscular blockade and consciousness are necessary for a safe tracheal extubation at the end of anesthesia.

Neuromuscular monitoring of depth is necessary in the morbidly obese to dose neuromuscular blockade antagonist to prevent residual paralysis, which affects genioglossus muscle activity during deep inspiration, causing retroglossal and retropalatal narrowing. These effects are particularly dangerous in morbidly obese patients because of the possible presence of obstructive sleep apnea syndrome.

The dose of sugammadex must be sufficient to affect the gradient between the peripheral and central compartments and more is required when repeated doses or continuous infusion of rocuronium.

3. Postoperative Management

Even if most patients are managed in ward, close supervision during 4-6 hour after surgery is mandatory. Postoperative continuous mechanical ventilation is necessary in less than 1% of patients; at risk are those affected by more severe hypoventilation syndrome or when hemorrhage or leaks are present. On the contrary, obstruction of upper airway and the limited functional respiratory capacity in morbid obese patients are common and facilitate hypoxemic episodes after bariatric surgery. To prevent it, reintroduction of continuous positive airway pressure is crucial. Also, a multimodal analgesia without opioid is preferable. Sitting bed patient position and early mobilization helps to fast-track process that will take 2-4 days.

1. Anesthesia Consideration and Management for Bariatric Surgery

The prevalence of morbid obesity has multiplied in the last fifteen years, and it has been associated with higher mortality in comparison with non obese population. Morbidly obese patients are at high risk of cardiovascular and respiratory functional overload related to varying degrees of metabolic syndrome. Most of the patients need bariatric surgery in an early stage of the disease to ensure low rates of mortality and morbidity are the standard. Because of that, a composite measure, which will involve combining serious complications, reoperations, and readmissions, is advisable to predict performance of the surgery. It is important to note that cardiovascular disorders are no longer a contraindication of surgery, and therefore, major postoperative complication and mortality can occur more frequently as morbid obese patient are accepted for any type of surgery.

Perioperative complications are related to the type of bariatric surgery. Restrictive procedures are not expected to have mortality, but all complication rates are 3.2%, and readmission rate is 4.3%. [1] For gastric bypass procedures, the complication rate is 16%, the readmission rate of 6.6% and mortality around 0.4%, which account intra operatively in 0.18% of patients. [1] Sleeve gastrectomy is performed in those high risk patients as an intermediate stage to definitive bypass procedure. Risk stratification predictors are: age, male sex, body mass index (BMI) and comorbidities [diabetes, obesity hypoventilation syndrome and heart disease]. [2-4]. Adverse anesthesia intraoperative events [multiple tracheal intubation attempts, sustained dysrhythmia and hypotension and hypercarbia] occurred in 0.9% of the patients. [3].

The whole bariatric population should be screened for obstructive sleep apnea (OSA) through the application of the Epworth sleepiness scale, Stop-band score or a clinical history of nocturnal snoring, morning headache or a large neck circumference, and if some of them are positive, a polysomonography study is mandatory as well as arterial blood gases for those patients affected by hypoventilation syndrome. Smoking cessation and pretreatment with non invasive positive airway pressure ventilation facilitate optimization previous to surgery. The patients with severe hypertension [those on two or more antihypertensive drugs], or history of acute heart disease should undergo cardiovascular evaluation from time to time, and a special attention has to be paid to those super obese patients (BMI > 70 $kg.m^{-1}$). Anesthetic treatment of morbid obese patients is a challenge, even to an experienced anesthesiologist, and to do that effectively some intraoperative key points have to be considered.

1.1. Safety in Airway Procurement at Anesthesia Induction

In order to facilitate oxygenation and the airway management, patients are placed in semi-sitting position and oxygen is administered to them to increase tolerance to apnea.

Because of neck fat accumulation, difficult tracheal intubation is present in around 10% of patients. [5-7]. For obese patients in ramped position, Airtraq™ have a faster tracheal intubation than the Macintosh laryngoscope. [8] It is a general opinion that, awake intubation should be indicated when any element of the triple airway maneuver [mandible advancement, neck extension, and mouth opening] is limited in patients with severe OSA. From our experience, [9] awake intubation is indicated when a limited mandible advancement is associated with a short tyromental distance (<6cm) and a Mallampati class 2/3/4. This conservative approach tries to reduce the "can ventilate and can't intubate" crisis, noticed in a range of 0.3-1.2% in our series of patients. [9] Awake tracheal intubation with videolaringoscope is a good alternative to fiber optical intubation [10-15]. The introduction of sugammadex, which is able to reverse quickly a neuromuscular blockade of any depth and ensure complete recovery of pharyngeal muscles [16], has displaced the use of succinylcholine for the rest of patients in whom a general anesthesia induction is planned. The outcome of that is a better oxygenation provided by rocuronium in comparison with succinylcholine [17] and a quicker recovery of spontaneous ventilation with rocuronium when high dose of both drugs are used. [18]. In a case report, the administration of sugammadex in a 'can't ventilate' scenario allowed return of spontaneous breathing before the development of hypoxia [19].

It is important to say that the reversal of neuromuscular blockade is not enough to obtain adequate ventilation, which also requires that the patient regain consciousness in order to avoid airway collapse caused by hypnotic drugs. [20]

The dose of propofol for anesthesia induction depends on the weight of the patient, consequently, some adjust to a large dose has to be made if ideal body weight is used to calculate the dose. On the contrary, neuromuscular blocker drugs can be dose by using ideal body weight. However, a rapid sequence induction is advisable for morbid obese patients.

1.2. Maintenance of Anesthesia during Laparoscopic Procedures

It was found that obesity caused a statistically significant increase in respiratory resistance and an increase in inspiratory pressure and a decrease in dynamic respiratory compliance when mechanical ventilation was started in laparoscopic surgery. In non obese patients, a definite plateau in the total exhaled carbon dioxide per minute was observed within 20 minutes from the start of pneumoperitoneum; on the contrary, the total exhaled carbon dioxide per minute increases during the whole surgery in the morbidly obese patients. [21] After disinflation, the total exhaled carbon dioxide per minute returned more rapidly to the baseline values in the non obese patients. [21]

In relation to ventilation strategies during surgery, there is some evidence that recruitment maneuvers added to positive expiratory pressure improves intraoperative oxygenation without changes in blood pressure; but, there is no evidence of any difference between pressure controlled ventilation and volume controlled ventilation. [22] A deep neuromuscular blockade facilitates ventilation and ensures an adequate surgical field facilitating the surgical procedure. From a clinical point of view, although neuromuscular monitoring is not widely used, it is therefore advisable to use it in all patients, being the train of four stimulus ratio [TOFr] at abductor pollicis the recommended monitor.

End-tidal of sevoflurane leading to a BIS value below 50 in 50% of the morbid obese patient has been observed in 1.6%, higher than that previously reported in non obese patients, 0.97%, and less than that reported in children, 2.8%. [23]. Both, desflurane and sevoflurane are suitable for maintenance of anesthesia, although. desflurane increased intestinal motility and decreased surgeon satisfaction compared with sevoflurane. [24].

Both, reversal of neuromuscular blockade and consciousness are necessary for a safe tracheal extubation at the end of anesthesia. On the basis of the awareness of residual neuromuscular blockade and its clinical implications, drug used during anesthesia should be considered in the morbidity risk analysis.

Neuromuscular monitoring of depth is necessary in the morbidly obese patients to dose neuromuscular blockade antagonist so as to prevent residual paralysis, that affects genioglossus muscle activity during deep inspiration, and causes retroglossal and retropalatal narrowing, with airway flow limitation; [25-27] changes also occur in swallowing as well as in inspiratory capacity and ventilatory response to hypoxia, which are reduced. [28, 29] These effects are particularly dangerous in morbidly obese patients because of the possible presence of obstructive sleep apnea syndrome. [30] Also at higher risk of upper airway collapse during the perioperative period, these patients should be fully awake and the neuromuscular blockade fully reversed before tracheal extubation is attempted. [31]

In contrast to anticholinesteric agent, sugammadex is able to reverse intense neuromuscular blockade, in a first step, and captures free rocuronium, leading to release of rocuronium from cell receptors. Even though the pharmacokinetic profile of sugammadex is affected by age and renal function, quick reversal (<2 minutes) occurs in lean patients after a sugammadex dose of 2 mg.kg-1 [moderate blockade] or 4 mg.kg-1 (deep blockade), either with propofol or sevofluorane for anesthesia maintenance. [32] The dose of sugammadex must be sufficient to affect the gradient between the peripheral and central compartments and more is required with repeated doses or continuous infusion of rocuronium. Overdoses will which result from using real body weight in morbidly obese patients in the standard calculations will be costly and ineffective in a high number of patients given the ceiling effect. Moreover, the safety and efficacy of sugammadex dose based on the ideal body weight has been questioned. Many morbid obese patients on sugammadex have different types of responses or reactions depending on the type of anesthesia, the total dose of neuromuscular blockade drug and time from the last dose of rocuronium.

Table 1. Dose of Sugammadex. Summary of data reported in Bariatric Surgery

	Dose mg/kg Real body weight	Time to TOF 0.9 [sc]	Time to tracheal extubation [sc]
Moderate blockade [T2]			
Standard Patients	2 mg/Kg	90 sc	
Obese Patient			
Van Lancker [33]	1.34 mg/kg	120 sc	255 sc
Van Lancker [33]	2 mg/Kg	128 sc	326 sc
Gaszynski [34]	1.29 mg/Kg	167 sc (265 sc)	-
Llaurado [35]	1.23 mg/Kg	113 sc (300 sc)	220 sc
Sanfilippo [36]	1.075 mg/Kg	151 ± 44 sc	
Sanfilippo [36]	2 mg/Kg	121 ± 21 sc	
Deep Blockade			
Standard Patient	4 mg/kg	90 sc	
Obese Patient			
Llaurado [35]	2.3 mg/Kg	167 sc (460 sc)	586 sc

1.3. Postoperative Management

Even if most patients are treated in ward, in a setting of fast-track surgery [40] close supervision from 4-6 hour after surgery is mandatory, because morbid obese patients carry significantly increased risk of extubation failure and are frequently associated with difficult airway management. Extubation failure is caused by loss of upper airway patency; edema, soft tissue collapse, and laryngospasm which are among the most frequent mechanisms of upper airway obstruction.[41]

Anesthesia induced atelectasis occurs in nearly all anesthetized patients; even if reversible after bariatric surgery, and hypoventilation syndrome determine respiratory complications in the postoperative period. [42] The reasons for abnormalities in regional ventilation produced during anesthesia and surgery are: hypoventilation due to pain or residual anesthetics, lung edema due to fluid overload and exacerbation of chronic obstructive pulmonary disease. [43] A clinically relevant fade in forced vital capacity is produced as a consequence of residual neuromuscular blockade. [44] Therefore, strategies to prevent respiratory complication or improve ventilation such as multimodal analgesia without opioid, sitting bed patient position and early mobilization, have to be implemented to help fast-track process that will take 2-4 days. [45]

Postoperative continuous mechanical ventilation is necessary in less than 1% of the patients; at risk are those affected by more severe hypoventilation syndrome or those with hemorrhage or leaks. Obstruction of upper airway and the limited functional respiratory capacity in morbid obese patients are the consequences of hypoxemic episodes after bariatric surgery. [46]

To prevent it, reintroduction of continuous positive airway pressure is crucial, as well as adequate reversal of neuromuscular blockade. [47, 48] Fewer episodes of postoperative oxygen desaturation [46] and less likely associated with X-ray results are consistent with postoperative complete reversal of neuromuscular blockade. [47, 48]

2. New Insights in Morbid Obese Patients' Management

A recent systematic review of medical journals concluded that there is no adequate information to make strong recommendations regarding appropriate selection of the obese patients scheduled for ambulatory surgery. However, the super obese patient (BMI>50 kg/ m) do present an increased risk for perioperative complications. [49] Patients affected by obstructive sleep apnea may be accepted for ambulatory surgery if they are able to use a continuous positive airway pressure device in the postoperative period and pain can be managed without opioid drugs. [50] A recent report indicates safety of performance of bariatric restrictive procedures in ambulatory regimen, 0.8 % of patients were transferred from the Ambulatory centre to a hospital and 3.6% of patients were readmitted within 30 days. [51] By using laryngeal mask instead of tracheal intubation, the requirements for neuromuscular blockade drugs were reduced and time to discharge the patients from both the postanesthesia care unit and the hospital also was reduced; [52] however, in two patients laryngeal mask had to be removed because of initial placement failed and in one patient a laryngospasm occurred after removal, which represent 8% of the failures.

For those patients with recurrent episodes of pulmonary thrombi embolism or with the contraindication of prophylaxis, the use of vena cava filters will remain controversial, even though its use continues to rise. [53] Thrombosis of vena cava related to filters is uncommon, but it may be present in at least 3% of the patients.

References

[1] American Association of Clinical Endocrinologist. The Obesity Society and American Society for Metabolic and Bariatric Surgery Medical. Guidelines for clinical practice for perioperative nutritional, metabolic and nonsurgical support of the bariatric surgery patient. *Surgery for Obesity and Related Diseases* 2008; 4: S109-S184.

[2] De Maria EJ, Portenier D, Wolfe L. Obesity surgery mortality risk score: proposal for a clinically useful score to predict mortality risk in patients undergoing gasgtric bypass. *Surg. Obes. Relat. Dis.* 2007; 3: 134-140.

[3] Marti Valeri C, Sabate A, Masdevall C, Camprubí I, Dalmau A, Gracia T, Koo M, Sanzol R, Suárez M, Montero A. Influencia del grado de obesidad en la morbimortalidad operatoria de la cirugia bariatrica. *Rev. Esp. Anestesiol. Reanim.* 2004; 51: 44-46.

[4] Maciejewski ML, Winegar DA, Farley JF, Wolfe BM, De Maria EJ. Risk stratification of serious adverse events alter bypass in the Bariatric Outcome Longitudinal Database. *Sur. Obes. Relat. Dis.* 2012; 8: 671-677.

[5] Brodsky JB, Lemmens HJM, Vierra M, Saidman LJ. Morbid obesity and tracheal *Intubation Anesth. Analg.* 2002; 94:732–6.

[6] Lavi R, Segal D, Ziser A. Predicting difficult airways using the intubation difficulty scale: a study comparing obese and non-obese patients. *J. Clin. Anesth.* 2009; 21: 264-7.

[7] Juvin P, Lavaut E, Dupont H, Lefevre P, Demetriou M, Dumoulin JL, et al. Difficult tracheal intubation is more common in obese than in lean patients. *Anesth. Analg.* 2003; 97: 595-600.

[8] Andersen LH, Rovsing L, Olsen KS. GlideScope videolaryngoscope vs. Macintosh direct laryngoscope for intubation of morbidly obese patients: a randomized trial. *Acta Anaesthesiol. Scand.* 2011; 55: 1090-7.

[9] Montealegre-Angarita MC, Llauradó-Paco S, Sabaté A, Ferreres E, Cabrera A, Camprubí I. Analysis of difficult intubation factors in bariatric surgery. Influence of the choice of neuromuscular blocker on the availability of sugammadex. *Rev. Esp. Anestesiol. Reanim.* 201; 60:434-9.

[10] Abdallah R, Galway U, You J, Kurz A, Sessler DI, Doyle DJ. A randomized comparison between the Pentax AWS video laryngoscope and the Macintosh laryngoscope in morbidly *Anesth. Analg.* 2011; 113:1082-7.

[11] Ydemann M, Rovsing L, Lindekaer AL, Olsen SK. Intubation of the morbidly obese patient: GlideScope vs. Fastrach. *Acta. Anaesthesiol. Scand.* 2012; 56: 755–761.

[12] Ranieri D, Filho SM, Batista S, do Nascimento P. Comparison of Macintosh and Airtraq TM laryngoscopes in obese patients placed in the ramped position. *Anaesthesia* 2012; 67: 980–985.

[13] Moore AR, Schricker T, Court O. Awake videolaryngoscopy-assisted tracheal intubation of the morbidly obese. *Anaesthesia* 2012; 67: 232–5. 23.

[14] Wender R, Goldman AJ. Awake insertion of the fibreoptic intubating LMA C Trach in three morbidly obese patients with potentially difficult airways. *Anaesthesia* 2007; 62: 948-51.

[15] Dimitriou VK, Zogogiannis ID, Liotiri DG. Awake tracheal intubation using the Airtraq laryngoscope: a case series. Acta Anaesthesiologica Scandinavica 2009; 53: 964–7. 5.

[16] Lee C, Jahr JS, Candiotti KA, Warriner B, Zornow MH, Naguib M. Reversal of profound neuromuscular block by sugammadex administered three minutes after rocuronium. *Anesthesiology* 2009; 110: 1020-5

[17] Tang L, Li S, Huang S, Ma H, Wang Z. Desaturation following rapid sequence induction using succinylcholine vs rocuronium in overweight patients. *Acta Anaesthesiol Scand* 2011; 55: 203-8.

[18] Sørensen MK, Bretlau C, Gatke R, Sørensen MA, Rasmussen LA. Rapid sequence induction and intubation with rocuronium-sugammadex compared with succinylcholine: a randomized trial. *Br. J. Anaesth.* 2012; 108: 682-9 22.

[19] Paton L, Gupta S, Blacoe D. Successful use of sugammadex in a 'can't ventilate' scenario. Anaesthesia. 2013; 68:861-4.

[20] Isono S. Obstructive sleep apnea of obese adults: pathophysiology and perioperative airway management. *Anesthesiology* 2009; 110:908 –21.

[21] Perilli V, Vitale F, Modesti C, Ciocchetti P, Sacco T, Sollazzi L Carbon dioxide elimination pattern in morbidly obese patients undergoing laparoscopic surgery *Surg. Obes. Relat. Dis.* 2012; 8: 590-4.

[22] Aldenkortt M, Lysakowski C, Elia N, Brochard L, Tramèr MR. Ventilation strategies in obese patients undergoing surgery: a quantitative systematic review and meta-analysis *Br. J. Anaesth.* 2012;109: 493-502.

[23] Zeidan A, Mazoit JX. Minimal alveolar concentration of sevoflurane for maintaining bispectral index below 50 in morbidly obese patients. *Acta Anaesthesiol. Scand.* 2013; 57:474-9.

[24] De Corte W, Delrue H, Vanfleteren LJ, Dutré PE, Pottel H, Devriendt DK, Van Rooy FH, D'Hondt M, Carlier S, Desmet MB. Randomized clinical trial on the influence of anaesthesia protocol on intestinal motility during laparoscopic surgery requiring small bowel anastomosis *Br. J. Surg.* 2012; 99: 1524-9.

[25] Eikermann M, Zaremba S, Malhotra A, Jordan AS, Rosow C, Chamberlin NL. Neostigmine but not sugammadex impairs upper airway dilator muscle activity and breathing. *Br. J. Anaesth* 2008; 101: 344-9.

[26] Herbstreit F, Peters J, Eikermann M. Impaired upper airway integrity by residual neuromuscular blockade. *Anesthesiology* 2009; 110: 1253-60.

[27] Eikermann M, Vogt FM, Hersbstreit F, Vahit-Dastgerdi M, Zenge MO, Ochterbeck C de Greiff A, Peters J. The predisposition to inspiratory upper airway collapse during partial neuromuscular blockade. *Am. J. Respir. Crit. Care Med.* 2007; 175: 9-15.

[28] Sundman E, Witt H, Olsson R, Ekberg O, Kuylenstierna R, Eriksson Ll. The incidence and mechanisms of pharyngeal and upper esophageal dysfunction in partially paralyzed humans. *Anesthesiology* 2000; 92: 977-84.

[29] Eriksson Ll, Sundman E, Olsson R, Nilsson L, Witt H, Ekberg O, Kuylenstierna R. Functional assessment of the pharynx at rest and during swallowing in partially paralyzed humans. *Anesthesiology* 1997; 87:1035-43.

[30] Schumann R, Jones SB, Ortiz VE, Connor K, Istvan P, Ozawa ET, Harvey AM, Carr DB. Best practice recommendations for anesthetic perioperative care and pain management in weight loss surgery. *Obesity Research* 2005; 13: 254-66.

[31] Frey WC, Pilcher J. Obstructive sleep-related breathing disorders in patients evaluated for bariatric surgery. *Obes. Surg*. 2003; 13: 676-83.

[32] Kleijn HJ, Zollinger DP, van den Heuvel MW, Kerbusch T. Population pharmacokinetic-pharmacodynamic analysis for sugammadex-mediated reversal of rocuronium induced neuromuscular blockade. *Br. J. Clin. Pharmacol.* 2011; 72: 415-33.

[33] Van Lancker P, Dillemans B, Bogaert T, Muller JP, De Kock M, Haspeslagh M. Ideal versus corrected body weight for dosage of sugammadex in morbidly obese patients. *Anaesthesia* 2011; 66: 721-5. 17.

[34] Gaszynski T, Szewczyk T, Gaszynski W. Randomized comparison of sugammadex and neostigmine for reversal of rocuronium-induced muscle relaxation in morbidly obese undergoing general anaesthesia *Br. J. of Anaesth.* 2012; 108: 236–9.

[35] Llaurado S, Sabaté A, Ferreres E, Camprubi I, Cabrera A. Sugammadex ideal body weight dose adjusted by level of neuromuscular blockade in laparoscopic bariatric surgery. *Anesthesiology* 2012; 117: 93-8.

[36] Sanfilippo M, Alessandri F, Wefki Abdelgawwad Shousha AA, Sabba A, Cutolo A. Sugammadex and ideal body weight in bariatric surgery. *Anesthesiol. Res. Pract.* 2013.

[37] Kotake Y, Ochiai R, Suzuki T, Ogawa S, Takagi S, Ozaki M, Nakatsuka I, Takeda J. Reversal with sugammadex in the absence of monitoring did not preclude residual neuromuscular block. *Anesth. Analg*. 2013; 117: 345-51.

[38] Grandjean B, Guerci P, F Vial, Raft J, Fuchs-Buder T, Bouaziz H. Sugammadex and profound rocuronium neuromuscular blockade induced by magnesium sulphate *Ann. Fr. Anesth. Reanim.* 2013; 32: 378-9.

[39] Murata T, Kubodera T, Ohbayashi M, Murase K, Adachi YU, Matsuda N. Recurarization after sugammadex following a prolonged rocuronium infusion for induced hypothermia. *Can. J. Anaesth*. 2013;60: 508-9.

[40] Carron M, Veronese S, Foletto M, Ori C. Sugammadex allows fast-track bariatric surgery. *Obes. Surg*. 2013; 23:1558-63.

[41] Cavallone LF, Vannucci A; American Society of Anesthesiologists Task Force on Management of the Difficult Airway. Review article: Extubation of the difficult airway and extubation failure. *Anesth. Analg*. 2013; 116: 368-83.

[42] Martí-Valeri C, Sabaté A, Masdevall C, Dalmau A. Improvement of associated respiratory problems in morbidly obese patients after open Roux-en-Y gastric bypass. *Obes Surg*. 2007; 17:1102-10.

[43] Tusman G, Bohm SH, Warner DO, Sprung J. Atelectasis and perioperative pulmonary complications in high-risk patients. *Curr. Opin. Anesthesiol* 2012, 25:1–10.

[44] Eikermann M, Blobner, M, Groeben, H, Rex, Ch, GroteT, Neuhauser M, Beiderlinden, M, Peters, JD. Postoperative upper airway obstruction after recovery of the train of four ratio of the adductor pollicis muscle from Neuromuscular Blockade. *Anesth. Analg.* 2006; 102: 937-4.

[45] Güldner A, Pelosi P, de Abreu MG. Non ventilatory strategies to prevent postoperative pulmonary complications. *Curr. Opin. Anaesthesiol*. 2013; 26:141-51.

[46] Sasaki N, Meyer MJ, Eikermann M. Postoperative respiratory muscle dysfunction: pathophysiology and preventive strategies.*Anesthesiology*. 2013; 118: 961-78.

[47] Ledowski T, Hillyard S, O'Dea B, Archer R, Vilas-Boas F, Kyle B. Introduction of sugammadex as standard reversal agent: Impact on the incidence of residual neuromuscular blockade and postoperative patient outcome. *Indian J. Anaesth*. 2013; 57:46-51.

[48] Llauradó S, Sabaté A, Ferreres E, Camprubí I, Cabrera A. Postoperative respiratory outcomes in laparoscopic bariatric surgery: Comparison of a prospective group of patients whose neuromuscular blockade was reverted with sugammadex and a historical one reverted with neostigmine. *Rev. Esp. Anestesiol Reanim*. 2014 Jan 8. doi: 10.1016/j.redar.2013.11.009.

[49] Joshi GP, Ahmad S, Riad W, Eckert S, Chung F. Selection of obese patients undergoing ambulatory surgery: a systematic review of the literature. *Anesth. Analg*. 2013 117:1082-91.

[50] Joshi GP, Ankichetty SP, Gan TJ, Chung F Society for Ambulatory Anesthesia consensus statement on preoperative selectionof adult patients with obstructive sleep apnea scheduled for ambulatory surgery. *Anesth. Analg*. 2012; 115: 1060-8.

[51] Billing PS, Crouthamel MR, Oling S, Landerholm RW. Outpatient laparoscopic sleeve gastrectomy in a free-standing ambulatory surgery center: first 250 cases. *Surg. Obes. Relat. Dis*. 2013; 17: S1550-7289.

[52] Carron M, Veronese S, Gomiero W, Foletto M, Nitti D, Ori C, Freo U. Hemodynamic and hormonal stress responses to endotracheal tube and ProSeal Laryngeal Mask Airway™ for laparoscopic gastric banding. *Anesthesiology*. 2012;117: 309-20.

[53] Sing RF, Fischer PE. Inferior vena cava filters: indications and management. *Curr. Opin. Cardiol*. 2013;28:625-31.

Index

A

accelerometers, 9
access, 37, 39, 44, 47, 91
accreditation, 36
achlorhydria, 21, 22
acid, viii, 19, 20, 26, 28, 29, 30, 32, 42, 43, 44, 46, 47, 52, 89, 100, 112, 113, 114
activity level, vii, 1, 3, 9, 11, 13, 16
ADA, 65, 68, 72
adaptation(s), 5, 6, 7
adductor, 130
adhesion(s), 37, 38, 88, 89, 102
adipocyte, ix, 85, 87, 88, 90, 97, 99, 100, 101, 102
adipokines, ix, 85, 87, 89, 90, 95, 97, 98, 102, 103
adiponectin, ix, 85, 90, 92, 93, 94, 97, 101, 102, 106
adipose, ix, 86, 87, 88, 89, 90, 95, 96, 97, 98, 99, 100, 101, 102, 105, 106, 107, 116
adipose tissue, ix, 86, 87, 88, 89, 90, 95, 96, 97, 98, 99, 100, 101, 102, 106, 107, 116
adiposity, 86, 102, 108
adolescents, 96, 106
adults, 14, 15, 17, 69, 74, 82, 86, 98, 102, 128
advancement, 122, 124
adverse event, 127
aerobic capacity, 12, 14
aerobic exercise, 12, 13, 17
age, ix, 7, 13, 22, 42, 43, 69, 70, 71, 72, 73, 74, 75, 77, 107, 114, 118, 121, 123, 125
aging population, 8
airways, 127, 128
albumin, 24
alcoholic liver disease, 49
alertness, 2, 4
alters, 23, 68
American Heart Association, 6, 14, 15
amino acid, 32
ammonia, 26
amniotic fluid, 115
anaerobic bacteria, 20, 29, 32
anastomosis, 20, 38, 40, 42, 46, 129
anastomotic leak, viii, 35, 39, 41, 43, 54, 56
anatomy, 44
anchoring, 47
anemia, 24, 25, 30, 96, 106, 112, 113
anesthesiologist, ix, 121, 124
anesthetics, 126
angiography, 101
angiotensin converting enzyme, 88
angiotensin II, 88
antibiotic, viii, 20, 24, 25, 27, 28, 29, 30, 32, 33, 39, 48
anticoagulation, 40
antidepressants, viii, 19, 22
antihypertensive drugs, 123
antioxidant, 88, 96
anxiety, 111
apnea, 51, 122, 124
apoptosis, 101
appendicitis, 113
appetite, 87, 88, 95, 104
appointments, 109
arterial blood gas, 123
artery, 46
asphyxia, 119
aspirate, 26
aspiration, 26, 43
aspiration pneumonia, 43
assessment, 13, 44, 54, 70, 74, 76, 79, 80, 94, 103, 129
asthma, 109, 110, 118
asymptomatic, 15, 22, 25, 28, 44, 52
ataxia, 25
atelectasia, viii, 35
atelectasis, 126

atherogenesis, 87, 90
atherosclerosis, 88, 89, 90, 99, 100, 101
atherosclerotic vascular disease, ix, 85, 86
autonomic neuropathy, 21
aversion, 111
avoidance, 42
awareness, 125

B

bacteria, 20, 22, 23, 24, 26, 28, 29, 30, 31, 44
bacterial fermentation, 20
bacterial overgrowth, viii, 19, 20, 22, 24, 26, 29, 30, 31, 32, 33
barium, 39
barriers, 110
behaviors, 16
benefits, 2, 4, 6, 9, 12, 61, 68, 119
benign, viii, 35
bile, viii, 19, 20, 23, 26, 31, 32, 43, 44, 113
bile acids, viii, 19, 23, 31
bioavailability, 97, 108
birth weight, 111, 114
births, 108
bleeding, viii, 35, 37, 39, 40, 47
blindness, 25
blockades, 125
blood, 6, 12, 24, 37, 38, 40, 48, 70, 88, 89, 97, 99, 109, 111, 124
blood flow, 38
blood monocytes, 99
blood pressure, 70, 88, 89, 124
blood supply, 48
body composition, 7, 13, 15, 16, 17, 105
body dissatisfaction, 59
body fat, 2, 7, 88, 90, 98, 102
body image, 53, 59
body mass index (BMI), ix, 7, 8, 9, 12, 13, 16, 22, 40, 42, 43, 46, 49, 50, 55, 57, 69, 70, 71, 72, 73, 74, 75, 76, 77, 78, 80, 82, 85, 86, 87, 88, 89, 90, 92, 93, 94, 96, 98, 101, 104, 105, 107, 108, 109, 113, 116, 117, 118, 121, 123, 127
body shape, 53
body weight, 12, 49, 76, 80, 88, 97, 98, 102, 124, 125, 126, 129
bone, 2, 5, 7, 97, 112, 119
bowel, 22, 25, 26, 31, 32, 37, 38, 43, 44, 45, 111, 113, 129
bowel obstruction, 43, 44, 113
brain, 88
Brazil, 24
breastfeeding, 113
breathing, 124, 129

C

calcium, 22, 45, 49, 110, 112, 113
caloric intake, 110
caloric restriction, 113
calorie, 17, 30, 69, 73, 112
calorimetry, 6, 8
cancer, 4, 58, 78
candidates, viii, 61capillary, 73, 111
carbohydrate(s), 17, 23, 45, 111
carbon dioxide, 124
cardiac surgery, 106
cardiorespiratory endurance, vii, 1
cardiorespiratory fitness, vii, 2, 3, 4, 6, 8, 12, 13, 15
cardiovascular disease(s), ix, 8, 51, 62, 81, 85, 86, 99, 101, 110, 116
cardiovascular disorders, 123
cardiovascular risk, 51, 58, 81, 82, 88, 100, 101, 103
Caucasian population, 99
cecum, 20
Celiac Disease, 21
cellulitis, 41
central nervous system, 88
central obesity, 98
cerebral hemorrhage, 112
cesarean section, 109, 114, 118
chemical, 40, 113
childhood, 109
children, 96, 106, 109, 125
cholecystectomy, 44, 56, 119
cholecystitis, 113
choledocholithiasis, 44
cholelithiasis, 43, 114
cholesterol, 51, 94, 113
chronic heart failure, 86, 98
chronic obstructive pulmonary disease, 41, 126
chronic renal failure, 41
cirrhosis, 49, 57
classification, 57
cleavages, 88
clinical diagnosis, 25
clinical disorders, 21
clinical presentation, 39, 42
cloning, 99
cobalamin, 23, 25, 32
cognitive function, 96
colitis, 28, 29
collaboration, 112, 115, 116
colon, 20, 52
colonization, 20, 31
colorectal cancer, 58
community, 100, 103
comorbidity, ix, 121

comparative analysis, viii, 61
complexity, 36
compliance, 9, 45, 68, 124
complications, vii, viii, ix, 8, 15, 19, 31, 35, 36, 37, 39, 40, 41, 42, 43, 47, 48, 49, 54, 55, 56, 62, 73, 78, 79, 81, 82, 91, 103, 108, 109, 110, 111, 113, 114, 115, 121, 123, 126, 127, 130
composition, 2, 7, 13, 16
compounds, 23
compression, 40
computed tomography (CT), 39
conception, 108, 109
conference, 57
configuration, 44
congenital malformations, 115
congestive heart failure, 41
consciousness, 122, 124, 125
consensus, vii, 1, 12, 52, 57, 58, 68, 108, 112, 114, 130
construction, 48
contamination, 26, 39
control group, 12, 22, 68, 70, 72, 74
controlled studies, 62, 68, 70, 79
controlled trials, 79, 80, 82, 103, 104
controversial, 44, 62, 90, 96, 127
controversies, 97
COPD, 41
coronary artery disease, 90, 100, 102
coronary heart disease, 4, 15, 101
correlation, 89, 97, 102
cost, 7, 41
counseling, 109, 111, 112, 115
c-peptide, 93, 94
C-reactive protein, ix, 85, 87, 94, 102, 117
CRP, ix, 85, 87, 89, 92, 93, 94, 96, 97
culture, 22, 28, 32, 103
culture media, 22
cure, 62, 68, 81
CVD, ix, 85, 86, 87, 88, 89, 90
cycles, 116
cytokines, 86, 87, 88, 89, 97, 98, 101, 102, 107

D

data analysis, 54
database, 70
DBP, 92, 94
deaths, 41, 110, 112, 114, 119
debridement, 41
defects, 38, 88, 108, 112, 113, 117
defense mechanisms, viii, 19, 20
deficiency(s), viii, ix, 19, 24, 25, 28, 29, 30, 31, 49, 86, 96, 97, 106, 110, 112, 114
deficit, 112
deflation, 111, 114
degradation, 97
dehydration, 48
Denmark, 22
Department of Health and Human Services, 15
deposition, 49, 95
depressants, 22
depth, 122, 124, 125
detectable, 93
detection, 108, 115
diabetes, viii, ix, 3, 4, 8, 19, 21, 25, 35, 41, 50, 57, 61, 62, 63, 64, 65, 66, 67, 68, 69, 70, 71, 72, 73, 74, 75, 76, 77, 78, 79, 80, 81, 82, 89, 90, 91, 98, 99, 102, 103, 105, 106, 107, 108, 109, 110, 115, 117, 123
diabetic neuropathy, 57
diabetic patients, 50, 100, 102
diagnostic criteria, 62, 75
diapedesis, 99
diaphoresis, 45, 111
diarrhea, 23, 25, 26, 28, 32, 33, 45, 49, 111
diastolic blood pressure, 94
diet, vii, 14, 17, 19, 28, 45, 47, 48, 52, 69, 70, 73, 74, 91, 104, 109, 111, 117
digestion, 23
dilation, 42, 48
discomfort, 47, 53
discordance, 73
diseases, 89, 101
disinflation, 124
dislocation, 47
disorder, viii, 20, 25
displacement, 113
dissatisfaction, 53
distribution, 15, 26, 98
diversity, 68
dizygotic, 109
dizziness, 45
dosage, 33, 129
dose-response relationship, 4
dosing, 29
drainage, 39, 41, 44, 48
drugs, 42, 69, 91, 124, 127
dumping, 45, 111, 113
duodenum, 20, 28, 44, 112
durability, 103
dysarthria, 25
dyslipidemia, viii, ix, 35, 51, 85, 86, 87, 90, 107, 110
dyspepsia, vii, 19
dysphagia, 42, 48

E

eczema, 118
edema, 25, 42, 43, 126
electrolyte imbalance, 49, 114
embolism, 41, 55, 127
embolus, 42
emergency, 56, 113, 118
emission, 50
encoding, 106
endocrine, 87, 95, 116
endoscopic retrograde cholangiopancreatography, 44
endoscopy, 46
endothelial cells, 99, 102
endothelial dysfunction, 90
endurance, vii, 1, 2, 5, 6, 7
energy, 2, 3, 4, 5, 7, 16, 46, 70, 73, 87, 106
energy expenditure, 2, 3, 4, 87, 106
enlargement, 44, 46
enteritis, 21, 25
environment, 109
environmental factors, 86
enzymes, 6, 20, 44, 96, 102
epidemic, 98, 116
equipment, 7, 36
erosion, 46, 113
erythropoietin, 94
esophagitis, 52
esophagus, 46, 110
ethics, 75
ethnicity, 7
evidence, vii, 2, 8, 9, 13, 22, 24, 39, 48, 58, 68, 71, 73, 78, 79, 80, 81, 111, 115, 119, 122, 124
evolution, 110
excess body weight, 78
exclusion, 73
exercise, vii, 1, 2, 3, 4, 5, 6, 7, 8, 12, 13, 14, 15, 16, 17, 51, 52, 68, 73, 75, 96, 99, 109, 115
exercise performance, 96
exposure, viii, 19, 52
extraction, 6

F

false positive, 26, 28
fascia, 47
fasting, 22, 26, 28, 62, 65, 67, 68, 69, 71, 72, 73, 74, 75, 76, 77, 78, 79, 91, 103, 111, 114
fasting glucose, 62, 65, 67, 68, 69, 71, 72, 73, 74, 75, 76, 77, 78, 79, 103
fat, 7, 8, 9, 12, 15, 16, 17, 23, 43, 45, 74, 87, 88, 92, 94, 95, 98, 112, 122, 124
fat intake, 45
fatty acids, 31
fear, 114
feedback inhibition, 90
fermentation, 20, 23, 26
ferritin, 92, 93, 94, 97
fertility, 110, 115, 116
fetal growth, 113, 114
fetus, 111, 112, 113, 114, 115, 116, 117
fever, 41
fiber(s), 6, 7, 44, 45, 122, 124
fibrin, 39
fibrinogen, 94
fibrinolytic, 88, 96
fibrosis, 49, 53
filters, 127, 131
filtration, 75
fitness, vii, 1, 2, 3, 4, 5, 6, 7, 8, 12, 13, 14, 15, 17
flatulence, 25
flexibility, 8
flora, 20, 31
fluctuations, 79
fluid, 23, 39, 41, 45, 47, 111, 114, 126
folate, 22, 24, 26, 45, 110, 112, 113
follicle, 108, 109, 116
food, 20, 22, 45, 46, 47, 88, 90, 95, 105, 112
food intake, 47, 88, 90, 95, 105
force, 2, 6
formation, 23, 42, 114

G

gallbladder, 113
gallstones, 43, 113
gastrectomy, 3, 21, 22, 37, 38, 39, 48, 49, 52, 53, 54, 55, 56, 57, 58, 62, 63, 64, 65, 66, 67, 70, 71, 73, 77, 79, 80, 82, 83, 91, 94, 106, 114, 119, 123, 130
gastric band surgery, ix, 86
gastric banding, ix, 3, 11, 16, 17, 22, 45, 55, 56, 57, 58, 62, 66, 67, 72, 75, 76, 77, 78, 79, 80, 82, 86, 91, 92, 95, 103, 104, 105, 106, 110, 115, 118, 119, 130
gastric bypass procedures, ix, 40, 70, 121, 123
gastric mucosa, 112
gastric outlet obstruction, 48
gastric ulcer, 113, 119
gastritis, 21, 22
gastroesophageal reflux, 51, 58, 110
gastrointestinal motility, viii, 19
gastrointestinal tract, 20
gastrojejunostomy, 41, 44, 55
gene expression, 102, 117
general adaptation syndrome, 5, 15

general anesthesia, 40, 122, 124, 129
genes, 88, 89
genetics, 86
Germany, 54
gestation, 109, 111, 114, 119
gestational age, 111, 114
gestational diabetes, 108, 111, 114, 115
glucose, viii, ix, 6, 12, 19, 22, 24, 26, 27, 28, 32, 57, 58, 63, 64, 65, 66, 67, 68, 69, 70, 71, 72, 73, 74, 75, 76, 77, 79, 80, 85, 86, 87, 88, 89, 90, 91, 92, 93, 94, 96, 101, 106, 110, 111
glucose tolerance, 12, 69, 75, 76, 90, 91, 110, 111
glucose tolerance test, 12, 69, 75, 76, 111
glue, 39
growth, 88, 105, 114
growth hormone, 105
guidelines, 14, 15, 28, 36, 40, 58, 69, 70, 75, 90, 108, 112, 117

H

H. pylori, 42
haptoglobin, 93, 96
headache, 123
healing, 48
health, vii, viii, 1, 2, 3, 4, 5, 7, 8, 12, 13, 14, 16, 35, 53, 91, 98, 102, 104, 106, 114, 116
Health and Human Services, 14, 15
health problems, viii, 35, 114
health risks, vii, 1, 3, 98
heart disease, ix, 86, 107, 116, 123
heart failure, ix, 40, 101, 107
heart rate, 6, 12, 13, 17, 109
heartburn, 48
height, 7, 48, 86, 98, 118
Helicobacter pylori, 21, 22, 42
hematemesis, 42, 46
hematochezia, 42
hematocrit, 40, 94
hemodialysis, 100, 102
hemoglobin, 50, 91, 94, 96
hemorrhage, 113, 123, 126
hemostasis, 58
hepatocytes, 96
hepcidin, ix, 86, 93, 97, 104, 106
hernia, 38, 44, 47, 56
hernia repair, 56
heterogeneity, 80, 108
hiatal hernia, 48
high fat, 117
high risk patients, 123
hirsutism, 52
homeostasis, 79, 80, 88, 94, 97, 106
hormone(s), 31, 98, 104, 109
hormone levels, 109
human, 15, 20, 31, 32, 87, 88, 89, 99, 100, 101, 102, 103, 105, 108
human chorionic gonadotropin, 108
Hunter, 117
hydrogen, viii, 19, 24, 26, 27, 28, 32
hydroxyl, 31
hyperandrogenism, 107
hypercholesterolemia, 90
hyperemesis, 113
hyperglycemia, 45, 62, 88
hyperlipidemia, 3, 57, 58, 108
hyperlipidemic state, ix, 85, 86
hyperparathyroidism, 112
hypertension, viii, ix, 3, 35, 51, 57, 76, 81, 85, 86, 87, 89, 90, 107, 108, 109, 110, 123
hypertriglyceridemia, 51, 89
hypertrophy, 7, 87, 100
hypoglycemia, 45, 111
hypotension, 45, 123
hypothermia, 130
hypoxia, 87, 90, 97, 106, 124, 125

I

ICAM, 99
idiopathic, 21
IL-8, 98
ileum, 20, 23, 112
images, 22
immune response, 88
immune system, 20
immunity, 89
improvements, vii, viii, 1, 2, 3, 4, 12, 13, 51, 53, 54, 61, 76, 80, 91, 106
in vitro, 101, 102
in vivo, 101, 102
incidence, vii, viii, 2, 22, 30, 35, 36, 39, 40, 41, 43, 47, 55, 75, 77, 78, 109, 113, 125, 129, 130
incisional hernia, 44
indirect measure, 24
individualization, 110
individuals, viii, 7, 8, 9, 12, 16, 17, 20, 22, 23, 24, 29, 35, 36, 51, 61, 86, 89, 90, 95, 97, 100
induction, 89, 99, 122, 124, 128
infarction, 116
infection, viii, 22, 30, 35, 41, 42, 46, 115
inferior vena cava, 37
infertility, 52, 107, 108, 116
inflammation, ix, 6, 46, 49, 53, 85, 86, 87, 88, 89, 90, 95, 97, 98, 99, 100, 101, 102, 103, 105, 106, 116

inflammatory bowel disease, 25
inflammatory changes, ix, 85, 86, 97, 98
inflammatory disease, 86
inflammatory markers, ix, 85, 97, 105
inflammatory mediators, 95
ingestion, 28
inhibitor, 22, 42, 87, 88, 90, 94, 100
initiation, 41, 75, 86
injury(s), 5, 8, 23, 32, 37, 38, 44, 49, 54, 95
inoculum, 44
insertion, 37, 38, 113, 128
insulin, ix, 6, 45, 52, 57, 70, 71, 73, 76, 85, 86, 87, 88, 89, 90, 91, 92, 93, 94, 96, 97, 99, 100, 101, 102, 103, 104, 105, 108, 111, 117
insulin resistance, ix, 6, 52, 85, 86, 87, 88, 89, 90, 94, 96, 97, 99, 100, 102, 103, 104, 108, 117
insulin sensitivity, 70, 86, 87, 89, 90, 91, 100, 101, 104
internalization, 97, 106
intervention, vii, 2, 5, 13, 17, 44, 69, 74, 75, 77, 81, 83, 91, 109, 114
intervention strategies, 17
intestine, 20, 22, 26, 28
intima, 100
intramuscular injection, 113
intravenously, 30
ron, ix, 45, 86, 87, 92, 94, 95, 96, 97, 103, 104, 106, 110, 112, 113
iron deficiency, ix, 86, 96, 97, 106, 112
iron transport, 106
irritable bowel syndrome, 25, 31, 32, 33
ischemia, 21, 37, 38, 42, 43, 46, 48, 54
isotope, 22

J

jejunum, 20, 28, 31
Jordan, 129

L

laceration, 38
lactic acid, 26
Lactobacillus, 24
lactose, 28, 45
lactose intolerance, 45
laparoscopic surgery, ix, 36, 54, 86, 122, 124, 128, 129
laparoscopy, 110
laparotomy, 44
large intestine, 20
laryngoscope, 124, 128
laryngospasm, 126, 127
later life, 62, 117
LDL, 51, 65, 94
lead, vii, ix, 19, 20, 25, 30, 37, 38, 44, 46, 47, 49, 86, 91, 97, 113
leakage, 44, 46, 56
leaks, 39, 48, 54, 123, 126
lean body mass, 3, 7, 9, 13, 92
learning, 41
left ventricle, 6
leisure, 2, 4
leptin, ix, 85, 86, 88, 90, 92, 93, 94, 95, 96, 97, 99, 103, 104, 105, 106
lesions, 23, 58
leukocytes, 86
life expectancy, ix, 86, 107, 110
life-threatening conditions, viii, 35
ligament, 5
lipid metabolism, 87, 88
lipids, 23
liver, 37, 38, 49, 52, 53, 58, 89, 97, 102
liver disease, 52, 58
liver function tests, 53
liver transplant, 37
liver transplantation, 37
longevity, 87
longitudinal study, 50
Louisiana, 17
low-density lipoprotein, 72, 89, 94, 96
low-grade inflammation, 96
lumen, 111
lysis, 38

M

macronutrients, 30
macrophages, 87, 89, 96, 99
macrosomia, 108, 109, 111, 114
magnesium, 130
magnetic resonance, 44
malabsorption, 20, 23, 25, 28, 29, 30, 32, 112, 114
malnutrition, 30, 49, 112, 114
mandible, 122, 124
manipulation, 37
mass, ix, 6, 7, 8, 9, 12, 16, 42, 49, 57, 82, 85, 86, 87, 88, 90, 92, 94, 95, 97, 98, 101, 102, 116, 117, 118, 121, 123
materials, 39
matrix, 98, 100
matrix metalloproteinase, 100
measurement(s), 2, 6, 7, 8, 26, 73, 74, 76, 79, 86, 98
mechanical ventilation, 123, 124, 126
meconium, 115

medical, vii, viii, 2, 19, 31, 35, 36, 40, 43, 47, 48, 50, 51, 57, 62, 68, 69, 70, 71, 72, 73, 74, 75, 76, 77, 79, 80, 81, 109, 110, 115, 127
medical history, 40
medically-complicated obesity, vii, 19
medication, 22, 64, 66, 67, 71, 72, 73, 75, 76, 95
melena, 40, 42
mellitus, 21, 57, 82, 86, 98, 103, 104
memory, 62, 81
menstrual cycles, 52
mesenteric vessels, 37
mesentery, 37, 38
meta-analysis, 3, 9, 14, 28, 51, 55, 78, 79, 82, 83, 99, 100, 103, 117, 118, 128
Metabolic, 3, 13, 27, 40, 45, 55, 57, 82, 104, 106, 119, 127
metabolic acidosis, 114
metabolic changes, 91, 104, 114
metabolic disorder(s), ix, 15, 107, 116
metabolic disturbances, 108
metabolic dysfunction, 86, 107
metabolic pathways, 88
metabolic syndrome, ix, 88, 89, 99, 100, 107, 108, 110, 115, 116, 121, 123
metabolism, ix, 16, 23, 32, 50, 68, 85, 86, 87, 89, 90, 97, 98, 99, 101, 103, 105, 106
metalloproteinase, 100
methodology, 8, 62
mice, 89, 90, 100
microcephaly, 112
micronutrients, 30, 45, 110, 112
microorganisms, 20
migration, 46, 48, 109
MMCs, 20, 22
models, 15, 108
modifications, 9, 47, 73
molecular weight, 40
molecules, 102
Moon, 119
morbidity, vii, ix, 1, 4, 41, 42, 54, 57, 85, 86, 110, 111, 113, 114, 118, 121, 123, 125
mortality, ix, 2, 4, 8, 14, 15, 36, 41, 42, 43, 54, 55, 56, 58, 62, 78, 85, 86, 90, 91, 98, 101, 111, 113, 115, 121, 123, 127
mortality rate, ix, 36, 41, 42, 43, 86, 115
mortality risk, 127
motility-altering medications, viii, 20, 28, 30
mucosa, 42
muscle mass, 12, 13
muscle relaxation, 129
muscle strain, 5
muscle strength, 12, 13
muscles, 122, 124
musculoskeletal, vii, 1, 14
musculoskeletal function, vii, 1
myocardial infarction, 42, 116
myopathy, 25

N

narcotic(s), viii, 19, 22
nasogastric tube, 43
National Academy of Sciences, 117
nausea, 30, 42, 43, 45, 46, 111, 114
necrosis, 87, 105
negative consequences, 112
neonates, 108, 114
neoplastic events, viii, 36
nephrolithiasis, 45, 49
nephropathy, 49, 81
neuromotor, 14
neurons, 88
New England, 15, 17
New Zealand, 61
nicotinamide, 99
nitric oxide, 88
North America, 15
nutrient(s), viii, 20, 30, 114
nutrition, 48, 112
nutritional assessment, 112, 115
nutritional deficiencies, vii, 19, 43, 110, 111, 114, 115
nutritional status, 32, 100, 105, 114, 115
nyctalopia, 25

O

obesity related co-morbidities, vii, 2, 3, 75
obstruction, 21, 42, 43, 44, 46, 48, 113, 114, 123, 126, 130
obstructive sleep apnea, 41, 51, 58, 86, 122, 123, 125, 127, 130
oleic acid, 31
omeprazole, 31
operations, 36, 37, 41, 42, 51, 54, 55, 57
optimization, 123
oral antibiotic, 24, 25, 33
oral antibiotics, 24
organ(s), 2, 7, 37, 87, 116
osteoarthritis, viii, 35
osteomalacia, 25
outpatient(s), 31, 103, 111
ovaries, 107
overlap, 25, 115

overweight, viii, ix, 13, 15, 35, 36, 53, 71, 86, 90, 99, 107, 108, 109, 110, 116, 117, 118, 128
oxalate, 49
oxidation, 6
oxidative stress, 89, 96, 105
oxygen, 6, 122, 124, 126
oxygen consumption, 6

P

PA changes, vii, 1, 4, 12
pain, 8, 26, 27, 42, 44, 45, 46, 48, 91, 126, 127, 129
pain management, 129
palpitations, 111
pancreatic cancer, 52
pancreatic insufficiency, 21
pancreatitis, 21, 114
paralysis, 122, 125
paralytic ileus, 44
parenchyma, 49
participants, 63, 64, 65, 66, 69, 70, 71, 72, 73, 74, 75, 76, 77, 79, 80
pathophysiological, 26, 102
pathophysiology, 23, 56, 90, 107, 128, 130
peptide, 92, 94, 100, 105, 106
perforation, 44, 119
perfusion, 6
perinatal, 109, 115, 117, 119
perioperative period, ix, 41, 86, 125
peripheral neuropathy, 25, 51
peripheral vascular disease, 41
peristalsis, 20
peritonitis, 44
permeability, 23
personality, 77
pharmaceutical, 73
pharmacological treatment, 115
pharynx, 129
phenotype, 4
Philadelphia, 14, 31
physical activity, vii, 1, 2, 3, 4, 5, 6, 8, 9, 11, 12, 13, 14, 15, 16, 17, 70, 86, 91
physical fitness, vii, 1, 2, 4, 5, 8, 13, 14
physicians, 81
physiology, 4, 15, 20, 30
placebo, 24, 28
plaque, 88, 99
plasma levels, 104
plasminogen, 87, 94, 100, 105
pneumonia, viii, 35, 40
polycystic ovarian syndrome, 58
population, viii, ix, 3, 12, 22, 35, 36, 51, 62, 75, 86, 105, 107, 108, 112, 113, 114, 116, 117, 119, 123
population control, 75
portal vein, 37
Portugal, 85, 107
positive relationship, 4, 9, 88
postoperative outcome, 59
preeclampsia, 108, 114, 117
pregnancy, ix, 107, 108, 109, 110, 111, 112, 113, 114, 115, 116, 117, 118, 119
preterm delivery, 115, 118
prevention, 13, 17, 56, 75, 87
principles, 5, 39
pro-inflammatory, 87, 89, 97, 99
prolapse, 46, 114
proliferation, 99, 109
promoter, 110
prophylactic, 55
prophylaxis, 40, 127
protective role, 89
protein synthesis, 7
proteins, 23, 96, 97, 107, 113
proteinuria, 108
proton pump inhibitors, viii, 19, 22, 52
psychological impact, viii, 36, 54
psychosocial stress, 59
public health, 14, 15, 96, 98
pulmonary disorders, viii, 35
pulmonary embolism, viii, 35, 39, 40, 41, 43, 55
pus, 41
P-value, 10

Q

quality assurance, 54
quality of life, vii, viii, ix, 2, 3, 8, 14, 16, 20, 24, 36, 53, 54, 57, 59, 86, 87, 91, 103, 104, 110

R

race, 7, 13
radiation, 21, 25, 31
RCP, 44
reactants, 87
reactive oxygen, 88
receptors, 89, 125
recognition, 115
reconstruction, 21, 22
recovery, 122, 124, 130
recurrence, 28, 29
regression, 7, 112
regression equation, 7
remission, 50, 51, 62, 63, 64, 65, 67, 68, 69, 70, 71, 72, 73, 74, 75, 76, 77, 79, 80, 91

renal failure, 41, 49
renin, 88
repair, 39, 44, 47, 48, 54
repetitions, 5, 7, 13
reproductive age, ix, 52, 107, 110, 115, 118
requirements, 40, 127
resection, 21, 26, 48
resistance, ix, 5, 6, 7, 8, 12, 13, 15, 28, 85, 86, 88, 99, 101, 124, 125
resolution, vii, 2, 4, 29, 51, 62, 70, 78, 79, 109, 110
respiratory failure, 40, 41, 43, 55
respiratory functional overload, ix, 121, 123
respiratory problems, 130
response, vii, 2, 5, 12, 26, 28, 45, 87, 91, 95, 105, 106, 125
restoration, 40
retardation, 114
retinol, 87, 100
retinopathy, 25, 81
rhinitis, 118
risk factors, ix, 6, 7, 14, 40, 43, 55, 85, 86, 89, 98, 101, 102, 104, 107
RNA, 101
root, 37, 38

S

safety, 36, 54, 81, 103, 125, 127
saliva, 20, 47
salts, 23
saturated fat, 73
saturation, 94, 97, 113
scleroderma, 21, 25, 33
secretion, ix, 86, 89, 90, 95, 103, 107, 112
sedentary behavior, 17
sedentary lifestyle, 86
self-esteem, 53
sensitivity, 26, 28, 90, 94, 102
sepsis, 39, 43, 113
serine, 90
serum, 22, 24, 27, 87, 90, 95, 99, 100, 102, 104, 105, 106
serum albumin, 24, 27
shortness of breath, 44
side effects, 29
signalling, 99
signs, 39, 41, 46, 54
skeletal muscle, 2, 4, 6, 7, 89, 101
skin, 41, 108, 111
skinfolds, 7
sleep apnea, 3, 110, 128
small intestine, 20, 22, 23, 26, 28, 29, 31, 32, 42
smoking, 42
smooth muscle cells, 89, 99
snoring, 123
solution, 110, 114
Spain, 35, 121
specialists, 12
species, 20, 24, 88
spinal cord, 25
spleen, 37
Spring, 99, 102, 104, 105, 106
stabilization, 49
starvation, 114
stasis, 20, 40
state(s), ix, 3, 5, 40, 58, 62, 79, 85, 86, 88, 89, 90, 96, 107
stenosis, 42, 48, 55, 56
sterile, 20
stimulation, 89
stimulus, 122, 125
stoma, 48, 95
stomach, 38, 39, 40, 42, 44, 45, 46, 47, 48, 91, 112
storage, 112
stratification, 40, 80, 123, 127
stress, 2, 5, 95, 130
stress response, 5, 130
stressors, 2, 5
stroke, 6, 86, 98, 116
stroke volume, 6
structure, 42, 110
subacute, 25
supervision, 112, 123, 126
supplementation, 30, 112, 115
suppression, 24, 47, 105
surgery-induced weight loss, vii, 1, 13, 105
surgical intervention, 40, 48, 77, 113, 114
surgical programs, vii, 1
surgical technique, 91
survival, 86
suture, 48
Sweden, 77, 109
sympathetic nervous system, 45
symptoms, 25, 26, 28, 29, 30, 32, 33, 42, 44, 45, 48, 52, 59, 113, 114, 115
syndrome, 20, 25, 30, 31, 32, 40, 45, 47, 52, 56, 58, 107, 108, 111, 113, 116, 122, 123, 125, 126
synthesis, ix, 86, 88
systolic blood pressure, 51, 72, 94

T

T cell, 89, 96
tachycardia, 39, 40, 44, 45, 111
Task Force, 101, 116, 130

techniques, viii, 13, 35, 37, 39, 41, 54, 91, 95, 97, 113
technology, 107, 116
tension, 38
testing, viii, 13, 14, 19, 24, 26, 28, 29, 32, 79
therapy, vii, viii, 19, 25, 27, 28, 29, 30, 32, 40, 41, 47, 48, 50, 51, 57, 61, 62, 63, 64, 65, 67, 68, 69, 71, 72, 73, 74, 75, 76, 77, 79, 80, 82, 104, 115
thrombosis, viii, 35, 37
tissue, ix, 2, 7, 38, 39, 41, 42, 43, 47, 86, 87, 89, 90, 97, 98, 100, 116, 126
TNF, 87, 88, 89, 90, 93, 94, 95, 96, 101, 102, 103
TNF-alpha, 101, 102, 103
TNF-α, 89, 90, 93, 94, 96
tobacco, 8, 41
tobacco smoking, 41
total cholesterol, 51
total energy, 12
toxicity, 29
training, 5, 6, 7, 12, 15, 17
transcription, 89, 97
transection, 37, 39, 47
transferrin, 93, 94, 97
transformation, 89
transfusion, 40
transitional countries, 96
transplantation, 49, 57
transverse colon, 38
trauma, 46, 108, 109
treatment, vii, ix, 19, 24, 25, 26, 28, 29, 30, 31, 32, 33, 36, 39, 41, 44, 45, 46, 47, 48, 54, 55, 56, 57, 58, 61, 62, 65, 71, 72, 75, 76, 80, 82, 83, 86, 91, 103, 104, 109, 110, 115, 116, 123
triglycerides, 6, 88, 117
tumor, ix, 85, 87, 94, 101, 102
tumor necrosis factor, ix, 85, 87, 94, 101, 102
turnover, 112
twinning, 118
type 2 diabetes, viii, 50, 57, 61, 68, 69, 70, 71, 72, 73, 74, 75, 76, 77, 78, 79, 80, 81, 82, 83, 86, 88, 99, 100, 101, 102, 103, 104, 110

U

UK, 117
ulcer, 42, 55
ultrasound, 44, 108, 117
United States, 15, 19, 41, 58
uterus, 113

V

vascular dysfunction, ix, 85, 88
vascular wall, 101
vascularization, 6
vasculature, 6
vasoconstriction, 88
VCAM, 99
vein, viii, 35, 37
ventilation, 122, 123, 124, 126
vessels, 39, 47
vitamin A, 25, 112
vitamin B1, 20, 23, 24, 25, 30, 45, 110, 112
vitamin B12, 20, 23, 24, 25, 30, 45, 110, 112
vitamin B12 deficiency, 20, 23, 25, 30
vitamin D, 25, 110, 112
vitamin D deficiency, 25, 112
vitamin deficiencies, viii, 19, 28, 30, 49
vitamin E, 25
vitamin K, 23, 112
vitamin supplementation, 45, 112
vitamins, 23, 112
volvulus, 119
vomiting, 38, 42, 43, 46, 48, 111, 114

W

walking, 4, 74
Washington, 1, 15, 19, 117
waste, 2, 5
weakness, 45, 125
weight gain, 13, 47, 86, 87, 95, 108, 109, 111, 115, 117
weight loss surgery, vii, 2, 3, 4, 8, 9, 12, 13, 50, 54, 55, 110, 129
weight management, 95, 115
weight reduction, 4, 101, 102, 110
weight status, 117
weight-loss surgery, vii, 1, 37, 39, 43
World Health Organization (WHO), 57, 86, 98
wound infection, 41

Z

zinc, 87, 102